Slowing the Churn in Direct Primary Care

(While Also Keeping Your Sanity)

Douglas Farrago, MD

Praise for

Slowing the Churn in Direct Primary Care While Also Keeping Your Sanity

Dr. Farrago has written an engaging, insightful book addressing the inevitable patient churn experienced by Direct Primary Care Physicians. Not only does his book provide a framework for evaluating the cause of, and your reaction to, churn, it is also loaded with many helpful strategies and suggestions for both slowing the churn and surviving it. Let's be honest, we all feel the sting of that churn, but this book will provide you with a structure to better address it.

Tiffany Leonard, MD
Deer View Family Medicine, Hatboro, PA

Dr. Farrago has been one of my mentors since 2016 when I first started exploring DPC. His hilarious and moving speeches inspired me to start my own practice, and I would not have been able to do so without his book, The Official Guide to Starting Your Own Direct Primary Care Practice. His new book, Slowing the Churn in Direct Primary Care While Also Keeping Your Sanity, is an enjoyable read, packed with tons of great advice for delivering amazing care to our current patients. As a brand new DPC doc, I know just how hard it is to get a new patient, so it's definitely important that I don't blow it with the ones I already have! Thank you, Dr. Farrago, for another great book about DPC.

Emily O'Rourke, MD
Fountain Direct Primary Care, Chesapeake, VA

Dr. Farrago's latest book does an excellent job of shedding light on the difficult subject of why patients leave your practice. It is a clear and straightforward look at the reasons behind patient turn over and also the steps that DPC physicians can take to help retain patients.

The book helps to empower physicians to take what can feel like a personal loss or attack and use that as a motivator for improving the business side of a DPC practice. It is a necessary read for any DPC practice, regardless of whether they are experiencing the strain of patient churn.

Kyle Hampton, DO
Arktos Direct Care, Fort Collins, CO

I needed this. I wish I had this 4 years ago when I first opened my DPC. This book should be required reading for every new DPC doc in the months before they open their practice. I had such an "I need every patient to survive" mentality to the detriment of my mental health. It took me a long time to be able to "let it go" for those abusive patients. I recall one that I would hear from multiple times a week. Eventually, she called me late on a Friday evening. She had a sore throat without a fever, just wanting me to call in some antibiotics. I politely explained it was viral and offered to meet her Saturday morning for a strep swab. While we were talking Saturday morning about a lot of issues besides her throat, she commented "I don't know why I even bother paying for this service. We could just use our insurance and go somewhere else." I did a happy dance when she finally quit a few weeks later. Your chapter on emails really spoke to me. It is still something I struggle with 4 years in. I loathe answering emails. My RN/wife basically has to force me to sit down and answer emails. I dictate my responses to her and she "cleans them up", typically making them more polite and less curt than my verbal responses. It feels to me that as soon as I clear out my inbox, it just fills back up by the next time I check it.

Thank you so much!

Matthew Hitchcock, MD
Hitchcock Family Medicine, Chattanooga, TN

Table of Contents

Acknowledgements

I want to thank my patients who have stayed with us because they trust in our care. I want to thank some of the patients who left me for giving me good feedback to make me a better doctor. I also want to thank some of the other patients who left me for….. leaving.

Thanks to Christine Creasey, my assistant/phlebotomist, for helping with the statistics for our office's churn and for doing such an incredible job in our office. I know a lot of patients stay with our practice just because of you.

I want to thank my wife, Debbie, for tolerating my insanity and listening to my whining. You are also an awesome practice manager and my mornings are always better when you are there.

Thank you, Allison Edwards MD, for sharing your churn data. It is good to have you as a peer and friend.

Lastly, I want to thank my group of DPC doctor friends who keep my spirits up and my head above water instead of underground.

Oh, one more thing, I have proofread this book about ten times, but I am not perfect. There are bound to be mistakes. Sorry.

SECTION ONE:
REFLECTION

Chapter One:
Introduction

This is my third book on direct primary care and I need to ask you one favor. Please make me stop writing. It's obvious that I have an issue and can't do it on my own. I need help. The problem is that there are just too many things we need to know in DPC and I just feel this compulsion to share what I've learned. Why? Because I am one of the earlier family docs who jumped into DPC and I kept making mistakes. So, here is another attempt of using my failures to educate others. I hope it helps.

This book is about churn or patient turnover. This is for those doctors, not only those in mature practices, but also for those newbies who are just starting out. Everyone needs to worry about losing patients. It is a blow to your ego when people are going out the door seemingly as fast as they are coming in. That is an over exaggeration but welcome to my paranoia. I am in my fifth year, as of this writing, and this churn still happens. Many DPC docs don't want to admit this because we are embarrassed. I know I am. I just decided to get past it and do the research to figure out why it happens and how to make it slow down or possibly stop.

So, why read a book about slowing the turnover of patients in your practice, or what is called churn, when you're a newbie and just starting your practice? Well, the truth is that you don't want to spend tremendous efforts getting patients to join just to have them leave you for reasons you CAN control. Turnover, or churn, has become one of the biggest issues in direct primary care, in my opinion. It takes so much time and so much personal investment to get patients onboard that you don't want them slipping through your fingers by not doing everything you can do to keep them. And it's hard not to take it personally because you get invested in their lives. You also feel that it's a slight against you. You think, "Am I a bad doctor?" or "Will I ever keep patients?" or "Why didn't I become a landscaper?"

I would say that the churn factor is the biggest bugaboos that I have in DPC. That and bear traps. Long story. Anyway, I don't care how many years I've been practice, it's been 23 and counting, it never gets easy for me. As much as I think I have thick skin there are many times where I am reminded that I don't and it really brings me down. That's when the ice cream comes out. And the candy. And the cake. What can I say? I'm human. We all are.

You would think that getting people to join the practice is the hardest part, and that is true in the beginning or when you first open up your DPC office. But at some point that part gets a lot easier. It reminds me of a Seinfeld episode where he went to rent a car and the rental person stated that they have his reservation but don't have the car he reserved. His argument was that anyone can take a reservation, it's keeping the reservation that is the hard part. The same is true with retaining your patients in direct primary care. I hate to say that almost anybody can get patients, but it's keeping patients that is crucial in making you successful.

I have done many lectures and keynote speeches on direct primary care and I am one of the biggest proponents of its possibilities. I have written two books on this subject alone and I am proud that they are the best sellers in this genre. I'm one of the founders of the Direct Primary Care Alliance. But you know what? All this means nothing when a patient leaves because she didn't like the tone of my email or she felt, after a year, that the cost wasn't worth it.

So, let's talk about YOUR cost for a second. Did you know that it's cheaper to keep the patients you have than to continue to market and onboard new patients? Did you know that this treadmill, where patients are leaving your practice, may drive you insane? It almost did me. Trust me, you need the information in this book.

All this being said, having some movement out of a practice is going to happen and is sometimes a good thing. You are sad when some patients leave. Some patients you really want to leave and some patients you can't get them to leave. The point of this book is to stop the avoidable churn of those patients you like and want to stay. This book is about turning that treadmill off so that you are not trying to replace the good ones who are exiting.

We are in the wild west of direct primary care. The ground rules and understandings of what works and what doesn't is still being figured out. Direct primary care is also not easy for some patients, and even doctors, to understand. Many people still do not know what we do or understand why we actually charge them personally for their care. The bottom line is that we are changing the culture of primary care. This sounds great but it means nothing when you're fighting to pay the bills. With that in mind, you don't want to give patients a reason to leave. Did you know that many early adopters are bored easily and have no loyalty? They are looking for mistakes so they can leave. This realization may make it easier for you to understand but it still sucks. At least you now know why a bunch of your first enrollees are going to be the ones who want to leave. That's just their personality.

I remember this one dude who joined when I first opened. I did EVERYTHING for him: tons of referrals to the right specialists, clarified a life-changing illness, got him on the right meds and got him tons of savings on labs. I was even texting with him in real time when he was in Africa. I knew something was up when one day while he was in our waiting area, a journalist came in to write about our practice and asked him if he would be interviewed. He said no. Hmmm. He was gone three months after joining. Early adopter. Experimenter. Got his money's worth and was out the door. Be well.

The point of telling you this is that there is nothing you can do to keep some patients. Others, however, just need to be reminded of how good you are. As weird as this may sound, you actually need to market to your own customers in order to slow the churn! Keeping your patients happy spreads via word-of-mouth which gets new patients. In other words, happy patients bring in other happy patients. So, you want to keep them happy and keep them bragging about the things you are doing. I'll show you some ways you can do that.

But patients will always be loyal to you, right? Yes and no. The times they are a changin'. Some patients are always going to be loyal, but the bottom line is that money has a lot to do with it. Many patients value a lot of other services more than what you are offering. Sorry to be a downer. You have got to realize that at some level they just will stop paying if they rationalize that it's worth paying the higher cable bill or the home food delivery service, etc. In other words, you CANNOT count on loyalty like the fee-for-services practices because they aren't charging monthly. Little secret: patients are really not loyal to them either.

This book is different from my other ones in that I'm going to specifically talk about doing those things that slow patients from leaving. The reason is that because once they leave they are probably gone forever. In fact, I'll teach you to never argue with anyone going out the door. I'll show you the right way to ask "why" they left. This book will talk about value, subscription fatigue, building trust, and doing the little things and the extra touches that may save you a lot of money and heartache in the long run.

I hope you enjoy this and share with others. I hope this saves you money and your esteem. I truly want DPC to take over primary care. It's time we be the change we want to see in the healthcare system. The only way to do that is to make DPC successful. So, here's to your success.

Chapter Two:
Analyze Why They Are Churning

I've chosen not to go too deep into data analysis on this subject of churn. For one, I am not really great at the technical side of statistics. I'm also not convinced that with such a small population it's easy to figure out. My research into other types of companies shows they have mega data that they can analyze from every touch point a customer hits with their company. It would be very hard to get that data for us and very expensive to analyze. What I'm going to show you is some information that fellow direct primary care doctor Allison Edwards, MD has for her practice and what we have for ours. We did ours by hand and so did she. The cost of hiring someone, or some company, to analyze this for you may be prohibitive. I don't know of any DPC doctor paying for this and I am not sure it would be worth it. I do think, however, that you can glean some information to figure out issues that you may want to address right now.

Right off the bat, I do have a problem with exit surveys that some experts recommend. Go ahead and try it if you like but this can get very personal and take a toll on your self-esteem. Early in my DPC career I would ask people why they left and I could not believe some of the responses I got. They had no problem being mean. My bigger issue was the out-and-out falsehoods from some of them. I used to get into a debate with them but that only made things worse. To be fair, these were patients I was busting my butt for who vanished with one single perceived slight. If you can handle negative feedback and want to use some type of exit survey, then good for you. For me, it was not worth it. That being said, my front staff person will call and ask everybody why they left and keep that information. She just doesn't tell me.

After five years, as of this writing, I have to tell you that the most common reason people leave is money. I think it is very hard for them to admit that they can't afford you or that they just don't want to pay you anymore. To defend their own egos, they tend to highlight or make up other reasons and state that is why they left. You need to be aware of this before you read into some feedback and beat yourself up about it. Also, human nature will dictate that you will focus on the meanest and most unappreciative patient. Or the worst part of their feedback. I was guilty of that. Please don't fall into that trap. To be honest, most patients are sad and apologetic when they decide to leave our office and commend us on how great we are. Don't let the very few change your perspective and then doubt this model. The DPC model has so many great advantages over the fee-for-service model that there is no way the unhappy ones will be getting that type of service anywhere else. Even any weak spots we have, that we should still work on, are small compared to any other model out there.

So, to be clear, we don't ignore what people tell us, but we have to keep it in perspective in order to feel good about what we're doing. Honestly, our intentions are always good and we truly try to help people. All DPC docs I have met have great hearts and are altruistic. If you pay attention to just the ill-fitting patients, then they may sway you into doing things you don't need to really do. And you know who those patients are. It's the ones who you thought were happy, who now complain on the way out, that throw us all for a loop and give us pause. We should, and do, pay attention to their complaints and feedback.

What to Use

There is a myriad of survey methods to use. I have Constant Contact for my newsletter which I will discuss later. I can use that for surveys as a one-time purchase for about $30. You can use Mail Chimp as well. It has a ton of other free services for surveying a small amount of people. So, you may need to upgrade if your practice is full. There are other services out there that will do more for you at a higher cost. It will even analyze certain things for you. As I said before, how much of that information is useable and worth the money is debatable. This is why we did it by hand as described below. That being said, the most important thing is getting some data and figuring it out yourself by trial-and-error.

Things to Analyze

The evidence, from my research into other industries, points in the direction of gathering at least some data to improve your service, which will absolutely slow the churn. How you want to do it is up to you. From what I can tell there are tons of things to look at:

1. What are your patients' demographics and is there something that correlates with a certain group?

    a. Can you figure out their persona? This is an archetypal representative of your customer based on various attributes, attitudes, and characteristics. You can use another survey to figure this out. For example, you can ask them what part of the practice they like the most? Least? And so on. This may help you drill down to find your perfect patient panel. For me, I have found that I definitely enjoy speaking and dealing with those who are motivated to exercise, eat right, etc.

2. Send out exit surveys

    a. I discussed this above. Be careful not to take it too personally and change your practice for a few recommendations from nasty people. As I stated before, I am convinced most people leave because of money and make up other reasons to save their ego. In summary, we don't do exit surveys. I have toyed with it over and over and decided against it. We just have our staff ask them why they are leaving and then collate that data.

3. Send out customer surveys to your present patients

    a. There are pros and cons to this. You definitely want to know what they love about your practice. It may not be what you think. It also allows you to truly understand your customers and what they want and don't want. For example, what are the pain points for patients? You also can figure out how customers are using your practice. Is it for acute visits mostly? Physicals? Follow-ups? Email? Texting? Phone calls? That being said, I have seen other DPC practice survey results and was blown away with the wishes and recommendations by patients. They want longer hours, weekend hours, night hours, and more home visits. Personally, I am not doing more house calls or working on weekends even if that is what they want. Mostly what these surveys prove to me is the concept of hedonistic adaptation (more on that later). Sorry, I am too old for these demands and want my own life too.

4. Loyalty Question

    a. They say this one question, more than any other, may really tell you a lot about how you are doing: "How likely is it that you would recommend Forest Direct Primary Care to a friend or family member?" There is a company that does this called the Net Promoter Score and you can do this easily with Mailchimp and their sister company, Survey Monkey. I have not used their system but you can find it at netpromoter.com. It uses this question to see which of your patients are loyal enthusiasts, which are just satisfied but may jump at any time, and which are unhappy customers. The scale is on their website but you may not need that to understand you have a problem.

5. Lastly, spend some time analyzing the flow of your office. Make sure you include your staff in this. Every office has some problem issues over and over again. Have you ever spent time trying to figure what those things are? For example, what are the bottlenecks for getting patients in? It could be how you schedule follow-ups or your physicals.

This chapter could go deeper if I was a techno geek. I am not. I suspect a lot of you aren't either. I think what I listed are the most salient points and the lowest lying fruit to pick off the tree. This book also goes through the issues I found in my practice, which I believe will be relevant to yours.

ANALYSIS

Example #1

Here is the data from Allison Edwards, MD from Kansas City Direct Primary Care. She was gracious enough to allow me to show this to you. She was also humble enough to expose herself in this way.

Pregnant	0	0.0%
"I'm not using you as much as I thought I would."	3	2.6%
Unhappy w/ care or service.	1	0.9%
Employee Termination (via employer account)	7	6.0%
Medicare Age-Out	8	6.8%
Substance Abuse	5	4.3%

Moved	12	10.3%
Confusion About Services (i.e. quit before being seen)	14	12.0%
"I got insurance."	32	27.4%
Death	1	0.9%
Too Expensive/Don't See Value	25	21.4%
Ghosted	22	18.8%
Clinic-Generated Termination	1	0.9%
Employee or Duplicate Chart	16	13.68%

There is a lot to unpack here. This also may not totally relate to you, but I would bet that it's pretty close. As you can see, there is a good amount of churn that happens in direct primary care. Hence, the reason I wrote this book. The most obvious thing this analysis shows is that people who get new insurance will jump. It's sad because this may be prevented if they are constantly reminded of how much money they are saving and the quality of service they are getting. The same goes for the second biggest issue which is the service is too expensive. The next two issues are "being ghosted", which means patients are not responding to the exit survey. This helps no one. The last one I see as a reason that people leave is the confusion about "what is DPC?" as they quit before even being seen. This is why we do meet-and-greets before people join.

Example #2:

Here is what we found over the last year in our practice:

Archival Stats for 2018

Clinic Generated Terminations	15	8%
Ghosted	0	0%
Too Expensive/Don't Use	9	5%
I got insurance	12	6%
Insurance changed	4	2%

Employee Termination	1	1%
Medicare Age	2	1%
Substance Abuse	2	1%
Moved offices	5	3%
Moved out of area/state	42	23%
Confusion About Model	0	0%
Deaths	1	1%
Finances	21	12%
College Student	5	3%
Residency	4	2%
Failed Payment	13	7%
Unknown reason	36	20%
Other	8	4%

Total amount of patients = 181

Single = 39

Couples = 20

Families = 24

Total amount lost or written off for 2018 = $4,925.00

Now for some math. We had 181 leave which when then divided over 12 months, which comes to 15 people leaving per month. This is a little confusing because it may be just three or four big families but I am not going to adjust for that now. This number is 2.5% of the practice each month. From what I can tell, from other subscription-based industries, this is pretty good. I also think it is standard for DPC but time will tell as others do this.

It's obvious that every DPC office could get better and we are no exception. It is nice to see that the biggest reason for leaving the practice is that they moved. The next biggest motivation is "unknown", which means we need to do a better job finding out why. "Finances", "failed payments", and "too expensive" are next and proves that money is ALWAYS an issue in DPC. Only 7% of ours left because they got insurance and 8% were terminated for many reasons that I will go into in later chapters.

So, what did we learn from this? Well, every practice is different. Sometimes you have no control over why people leave. Sometimes you do and our office found that we need to dig in and find out what that "unknown reason" is for some of our churn. My guess is that it isn't a flattering answer. The finances or money issue is real for some patients and embellished by others. Remember, you can't save them all. If you can cut your churn rate in half then you will be much more profitable and less stressed. It also makes it easier to get rid of some other patients who aren't a fit.

Chapter Three:
Not All Patients Are For You

This may not be intuitive, and actually may seem to be counter-productive to slowing churn but knowing that all patients are not for you is key to your success and happiness. I understand taking "all comers" when starting out in DPC, in order to make a living, but over time you'll learn that this habit will break you. It will crush your spirits, make you cry into your pillow at night, and may even cause incontinence. I may have exaggerated the last one (as far as you know). Back to my story. Be careful about who you invite into your personal sanctum or happy place. It has nothing to do with their insurance or their illness. It has nothing to do with socioeconomic status. It is about working with people you get along with. They are your partners in their health. For you to have an impact on them they need to buy into what you are selling. So, if you are not into "integrative" medicine or cannabis then maybe you don't want those patients asking for this to join. Or, if you aren't really keen on taking on poorly motivated patients (diet, exercise, taking their meds) then why torture yourself? Or if you just know that they are jumping in to test the waters or to use you for a month then why go through all that effort? This is why, in my office, I do a meet-and-greet for every family before we invite them to join. We tell them that this visit is to see if this practice is the right fit for them but that street goes both ways. The bigger question may be are they the right fit for us?

Some DPC docs are told to imagine the perfect patient via an avatar. This is also called a "persona" in the last chapter. They picture their age, sex, body type, attitude, job, weight, hair color, etc. and then build their marketing plan around that. This sounds great but family practice is so diverse that this was just hard for me. Let's reverse this. Let's think about patients you don't want. For me, I have no trouble with challenging patients who have chronic problems. I do have issues with patients who are not open-minded, who want me to find a miracle cure, who want me to order what their chiropractor wants, and on and on. If I find, at their meet-and-greet, that they are rude to me or my staff or are extremely skeptical of the whole DPC concept then there will be problems later on. Some people just have a look on their faces at the meet-and-greets as if it is a bother to be there. This is so weird to me because they called us. I am blown away by how often this happens. They act as if the office smells like a roomful of farts. It doesn't. Seriously, it doesn't. I used to do the incredible sell to these people to convince them how great DPC is. You know what? Their scowl never came off their faces and they never joined anyway. Those people are not for me.

Let me give you some examples. I've had patients who are adamant about the toxicities of vaccines. During my initiation, before they join, I will explain my pro-vaccine stance and if they are skeptical to a point of being argumentative then they are not going to work in my practice. This is not to say that I don't have non-vaxxers in my practice, as I believe everyone should still be allowed a medical home, but I am not going to have an argument with someone on every visit. It also shows that they are very easily duped into internet rabbit holes and that is worrisome to me. I've had patients come in extolling the virtues of cannabis or CBD oil and when I explain to them that it is no panacea they get turned off. This is another red flag. I have had patients who are on tremendous amount of narcotics and I explain that I'm open to prescribing them but will try to hopefully wean them off and will definitely not accelerate their use. If they get bothered by this, then they are not going to be invited to join. I've had patients who want me to play CSI and discover their missing allergy or vitamin that would fix all their ills. I explain to them that I will do the best I can but there are no guarantees and that all I can do is be honest and open. If they are bothered by that then I don't take them on either. I've had patients who are just rude and state they hate doctors. Those patients aren't going to stay so I don't take them on. I've had patients who want to get everything done in the first few weeks, which tips me off that they're not here for the long run and are going to jump. These people are not asked to join.

You can find any way you want that works for you. And I am not telling you that the patients who don't fit into my practice won't fit into yours. This is a judgment call and I am not judging you. I am just trying to give you tools, or make you think about creating tools, that will work for you. Another way to think about this is to ask yourself, which patients in my past were poor fits? Maybe it's the ones who were cynical that you had to sell harder into joining your practice? Maybe it's those who were just miserable EVERY TIME you saw them and there was nothing you could do can to stop them from draining all your energy?

Try this test. For your next troublesome patient, ask yourself, "Knowing what I know now, would I still ask this patient to be in my practice?" If the answer is no, then think about firing them (see next chapter) but also think about the avatar/persona of this patient and what "tells" there can be for other patients. Start by getting a pen and paper and writing things down. Ask your spouse. Ask your staff. Do a test of going back in time and picturing your worst patients that you fired or who left you. What was the common theme? Or was there any particular theme? If you have been in a DPC practice for some time, you can go back and analyze the ones who have left you. Ask yourself which ones made you happy when they left and what were the commonalties. Or, do a two-week survey and during this time mark down names of people that you wish were gone. Why? What are they doing that irks you? Can you make a change so that you don't invite those type of people again? All this could have been easily stopped right at the meet-and-greet.

This is not to say that you will be perfect at this. I am certainly not. Some of them you never see coming. Even at my stage of the game I still get burned. I recently had a couple come in who was never happy with their past doctors. That should've been a red flag. When asked for their records they said it's not worth it as they felt it would will be incorrect, whatever that means. But once again my ego took over and I thought to myself, "I'm different. I'm a great doctor and I can help them". It turned out to be an easy sell to have them join the practice but in reality, it was not to be. Oh, they joined, and I did my dog-and-pony show to make them happy, but it never worked. The woman never stopped talking or complaining at each visit. I was cut off on every piece of advice I gave. Eventually, as I thought I was making progress in understanding their issues and getting them healthier, they quit the practice. Their complaint was they "couldn't get a word in edgewise" and "I was not the doctor" they thought they wanted. Shame on me. But like water off a duck's back, I had to let it go and learn a lesson from it. Be well.

There are no easy answers for this. This is a process for you to work on and to work with your staff on. Many times, I am open to taking challenging people, but if my staff tells me that this is not going to work for our office then I need to heed that advice. Sometimes I override them but most of the time they end up being right. The point of this section is that you have to work on this and make it a priority. You have to spend the energy finding out which patients are appropriate for you and which ones are going to be a problem. Sure, you want to make money, but in the long run it's probably not worth it. Hopefully you'll get to the point where you're 90% on point of who you want in your practice and who you allow to join. But most of all, make sure your office doesn't smell like a roomful of farts.

Extra Nugget: I just saw a patient for over an hour. I could not make her happy. I knew she had a million problems but took her on anyway. She left with a scowl. Instead of being greedy (and keeping her money) or letting my ego take charge ("I can make her like me"), I sent this email the next day:

Dear _____,

Christine told me that she felt you were not happy with your visit. I am sorry if you felt that way. There is a lot to process there. As I said in our meet-and-greet, all I can do is work hard and be honest. My style isn't for everyone and that is ok. If you are having second thoughts, then I understand. We will return all your money at this point if you want to go back to your last doctor.

Be well,

Dr. F

It felt so freeing to write this. It gave me a skip in my step for the rest of the day.

The next day she emailed back stating that she wanted to stay. This time, the only thing that skipped was my heart. At least I tried.

Chapter Four:
What About the Bad Ones
You Have Now?

O nce again, I am throwing you another curveball by writing a section on how to get rid of patients. Well, as I said in the previous chapter, you need to figure out who your best patients are so that you can dissect how you can keep them and get rid of the others. There are patients who are just a bad fit for you. These people will drain you of your energy and will burn you out as a direct primary care doctor.

If you have these "bad fit" patients, then you need to start getting rid of them. In no way am I saying that you should discriminate against any patient because of their medical or financial problems. I give away 10% of my care for free so I can't be accused of ignoring the latter. For the former, sometimes the most medically challenging patients are the most fun to work with. And in no way am I asking you to discriminate against any patient due to their race, gender, beliefs, or religion. But there are certain patients who can drive you nuts and that's a personal decision for you. Everyone has them and you're taking abuse you don't need to take and that will eventually sour you on the whole profession.

Now onto the most important part. You need, at some point, to think of your practice as a bonsai tree. You have to constantly analyze and prune the tree so that it eventually looks how you want it to. I have heard so many other direct primary care doctors online complain how their practices, even small ones, have gotten out of hand. It can happen to the best of us. This does not mean you can't fix it with some of the recommendations I give later in this book. But there are certain patients that just need to go. So how do you do that? I recommend the "Farrago Method of Firing". Here is how you do it.

If a few of your patients are the type that are abusing your service for non-issues and it affects the care you give others by taking needed appointment slots, then the best way to start the removal process is to just slow down on your responses. Many of these patients just need training or a detailed explanation of your expectations. This could be your fault and I explain that in another chapter. In fact, they just may not understand your capabilities or don't realize that they are not the only patients in your practice. For some, however, it doesn't matter what you do, nothing changes their behavior. For those who still are extremely demanding, and you cannot maintain this pace of access, then I recommend you pull back on how quickly you answer their email/texts or get them in and just see how they react. A small percentage will get it and that is part of the training process. For others, though, they will eventually start complaining and that is your sign that nothing will ever please them. So, go with it. As you pull back on your responses or delay your communication/ access, they may get more belligerent. When you have had enough, you schedule them to come for a visit just to go over their concerns. That should be your final visit with them. On that encounter you listen to all their complaints and then you agree with them 100%. I say things like "I see where you're coming from and I agree that I am not meeting your expectations. There is no reason you should pay for a service when I'm not coming through on what you feel you need. Here is what I'm going to do. I don't feel I can meet the needs that you demand at this time which is not your fault. It's just that I am unable to do it. Therefore, I'm going to return last month's membership fee and then give you thirty days free to cover you while you find somebody who can meet your needs."

But does giving them a month back of membership feel like I am paying to get rid of them, you ask? Yes. It's worth it. It's like paying terrible renters $500 to leave your unit because they are causing so much damage. You win in the long run. Lick your wounds and move on.

The key here is you have to make it seem like it's all your fault. You want to take the high road and you don't want them to leave mad. This doesn't always work, and many will still fight you just to stay. Do not give in! You will want to, but your mind has to be made up before they come in. Most of these patients will just try to convince you to switch your ways and coddle them some more. Your job is to hold your ground and not acquiesce, no matter what. They may start to get angry and you still need to hold your ground. Wish them the best, end the meeting, and then move onto the next patient or out of the room. No matter how much they complain that they still want to stay with the practice, do not let them! Your greatest day of freedom is the day you realize they're no longer with you. It won't feel like that immediately. You will feel bad. You will feel torn. It will sting for a few days, but it is so worth it. I really can't tell you how much this has helped me. I haven't done it much, maybe a half dozen times over the years, but the feeling a month later, when the noise is over, is glorious.

When you let the abusive patients go you can now spend time with the patients who you really like and appreciate you. Those are the ones you feel great about helping. Those are the ones who make you realize why you became a doctor in the first place. With the "negative avatars" gone you get to concentrate on being of service to the majority of your patients and that will probably be the greatest thing that has ever happened to your office.

Okay, I know this chapter comes off mean but I don't want it to. We still can't hide our heads in the ground. Like I said, some patients who are the bane of my existence, may be perfect for you. And I don't mind doing hard work or seeing patients when they really have problems especially when they are appreciative. I have had patients who seemed fine at the meet-and-greet who subsequently unveiled their true, and sometimes borderline, personalities within their first month and I get pissed at myself for missing that. But I will keep learning because I refuse to be abused like that. This is not how I want to practice medicine. I need to practice medicine with patients who I can enjoy being with and who I feel that I can help.

On to more important things.

Chapter Five:
Whipped Cream

Okay, we talked about not taking and/or getting rid of the "wrong" patients. Now let's talk about your office in general or at a macroscopic level. Would you say it is awesome? Perfect? Seamless? A beacon for other DPC offices to emulate? I ask this because before you really worry about churn you first need to know one thing and that is YOU CANNOT PUT WHIPPED CREAM ON DOG SHIT. I am taking a liberty here and using some information from my first book because even if you read it you need to remind yourself of these points. You cannot market your new DPC office without having a great practice. We all know you don't get a second chance at a first impression, but every other impression counts almost as much. In other words, if you're not doing great work, then you will lose patients almost as soon as you get them. So be great at what you do. You need to underpromise and overdeliver. As Steve Martin famously said, "Be so good they can't ignore you". Do not gloss over this and worry about churn unless you know your office is dialed in on every part of giving great care. The first step in figuring out why patients are leaving is to assess your clinic to see how you can get better.

Give Better Service

Service is one of those things doctors don't truly understand, especially those coming from fee-for-service model. I know I didn't. Usually we are so overwhelmed in patient care that we don't care about it. I get it, you went to medical school. You are smart and knowledgeable and that is the foundation of being a good doctor. But are you personable? This is beyond the basics of history taking and doing a physical exam. This is about running a business. Are you actually giving patients the time they need to talk? Are you making eye contact or actually listening? I know you can come to a diagnosis and help them out but this is just the starting point to a DPC practice. The history taking, the exam and the diagnosis are the reasons you have all those medical school loans. This, unfortunately, is the easy part. Now for the harder part. It's about doing the little things that count so please read my first book where I go into more detail on this, but here are some quick questions:

- Is your parking lot big enough?
- Does your office smell good?
- Is it clean?
- Is there nice music playing?
- Is it easy to call the office and talk to a human?
- Is it easy to get in touch with you?
- Is your front desk person and/or other staff friendly and personable?
- Do you follow up on issues for patients?
- Do you know your patients?

You need to thoroughly analyze the patient's experience from the moment he/she joins, sets up his/her first appointment, what goes on while in the office and his/her experience when leaving the visit. Fix your service before worrying about churn.

Build Trust

Part of your job, as a doctor, is building trust with the patients. They need to trust that you care. They need to trust that you listen. They need to trust your recommendations. You do this by listening, being empathetic and giving them time. By giving them much more value than any alternative office out there, you are locking them into staying with you. Honestly, right now it is like shooting fish in a barrel because the fee-for-service models out there are so poorly managed that it's very easy to beat them. But what if a DPC practice is opening down the block from you? Can't happen? Well, it's happening to me right now as I write this. Our service blows any FFS away. Now I have to make sure I am as good as or better than the new hybrid DPC opening up. Don't worry, I've got this, even though he is undercutting my prices. That being said, money does funny things to people/patients. You need to make sure you are doing some things so well (service, care, intangibles, etc.) that your patients are able to justify in their heads that you're worth that monthly fee that you are charging them. It doesn't really matter if you can show them you still save them money with their high deductible plans. They just see that monthly fee coming out of their accounts and they are saying to themselves, "Hmmm, is it still worth going there?" Your goal is to build a connection with these patients so that they always answer yes. Your practice cannot be a luxury they can do without. Your skills, your service and your caring need to make an impact in their lives. By being their trusted doctor, you are reinforcing and reminding them why they are paying for you. This is one way to prevent what's called subscription fatigue, or the phenomenon where people just get tired of seeing that monthly fee come out of their credit card or bank.

The Wow Factor

In my old practice, before doing direct primary care, I had a partner who would do what we called the "Johnny Show". This was his pretend Vaudeville routine that he would go through in order to make patients happy. We would laugh later, while eating lunch together, as he explained how he basically tap danced into the room, put his smiley face on and "acted" his way through the visit to make patients happy. Was he crazy? Yes, but not because of this. We, in DPC, also need to do a "show", but it has to be authentic.

There has to be a wow factor in your office. For me it is the office itself, which is usually empty for patients while they are here for a visit. Kim Kardashian doesn't even have this. In fact, if you've ever seen any of those shows where one of them is at a doctor's office there are always other patients in the office with their faces blurred. (This does not mean I watch their show. I have seen a few but..... okay, I'll stop. I've already said too much). Our other "wow" factors include us knowing the patient's name and asking about their family, offering water or coffee, and giving them the time they need while they are here. I also do a few more things that I will mention in later chapters. Superficial, you say? Maybe. But don't underestimate its significance.

There are a few caveats to this. I mentioned being authentic, so you really don't want to put on an act. You just want to be the best you. Leave your last visit behind you. Leave your worries and home issues at the door. Patients don't need your baggage. Be kind. Be nice and show you are there for them. Be personable so you don't become an energy drain on them. Take your time and be the doctor that you would want to see if you were a patient.

All this has to be consistent from the first time you see the patient and throughout their membership, which will hopefully be a long time. That being said, the mantra in the subscription service world (from reading the books on other industries) is that you better start out strong. You only have a short window to prove yourself. You want to start out with a quick win so your patients are motivated to stay with you. They need this wow experience in the beginning, at least, or some outcome that blows them away. You don't want to screw this up or you may lose them. They say the first 90 days is critical so pack a ton of value in each visit and add other value items as described later in this book.

Be Remarkable

If you want people to remember you for anything then you need to be remarkable. Be a great family doctor with a large bag of tools to help your patients. We are trained so well to handle so much, so use it all. Sure, you can handle an ear infection but what about other niches you are good at? For example, are you knowledgeable about lifestyle medicine where you are proactive in education about diet and exercise? What other areas are you great at that you can work with patients on? Supplements? Working with alternative modalities or your relationships with other practitioners in acupuncture or a Cross Fit gym? Maybe you do aesthetics or PRP injections? It doesn't matter what it is so much as you are offering other great things that make you and your practice great. So, I would recommend that you start listing how your practice is remarkable. Spend some time in creating this list. You can even use it later for marketing, but it also may show you some areas where you are deficient and can get better. Remember, just like in romantic relationships, never take your patients for granted. Never stop adding value. They crave new things to capture their attention and you're there to give that to them, to a certain extent. I know this sounds crazy but if you don't keep trying things then the relationship may become stagnant and you eventually will lose some patients. Keep it fresh, baby!

Clear Expectations

One way to prepare patients for their membership is to give them a clear understanding of what you do. Some people thought they could contact me any time, any day and have me come to their house and treat them. Some people thought they could be seen immediately anytime they wanted. I mean even the President doesn't get that type of service! But maybe it is not all their fault. It's about setting boundaries, and maybe more importantly, setting expectations. One way you can do this is to send them an initial email with a roadmap about the upcoming year after they join. Here is something we do with that communication:

a. Explain the practice.

b. Explain why we want them in for a physical once a year.

c. Explain why our deep dive labs are awesome and cheaper.

d. Explain how important follow up visits are for chronic medical issues.

e. Explain why we want to talk to them about lifestyle changes including exercise and diet and that we will try to keep them accountable.

f. Tell them that we offer large group lectures regularly and they will benefit greatly by coming.

g. Mention that we have a yearly holiday party as a thank you to our patients.

h. Mention that we get the free mammogram van to come right to our office as a benefit to our patients.

All this comes in our initial "welcome to the practice" email, which is located in Appendix C. You can do it any way you want. I have even toyed with making a video on how to use our practice/service. Whatever works for you is fine, but all of this sets the groundwork for a great working relationship. It gives realistic expectations about your practice so that patients aren't surprised or underwhelmed. You may also want to add information about boundaries or guidelines to your regular newsletter so patients are constantly reminded. This prevents uncomfortable situations later on.

I can't tell you enough how important all of this is. Yes, you want a thriving DPC practice, but you cannot collect $200 dollars without passing Go and you cannot create and build some loyalty, which slows churn, without making sure your practice isn't dog shit. Only after that can you add whipped cream to a beautiful pie that patients want to eat from. Now who is ready for dessert?

Chapter Six:
Hedonistic Adaptation

D irect primary care is also fighting an inherent weakness in human nature. People get used to incredible things and forget how good they have it. I am not innocent of this. We are all guilty in some way or another. The problem is in how it affects our practice.

In the book *A Guide to the Good Life: The Ancient Art of Stoic Joy* by William Irvine, he talks about Stoic philosophy and part of it is about trying to be content. In order to be content, we have to appreciate what we already have. The author says "We humans are unhappy in large part because we are insatiable; after working hard to get what we want, we routinely lose interest in the object of our desire. Rather than feeling satisfied, we feel a bit bored, and in response to this boredom, we go on to form new, even grander desires." Basically, we start taking things for granted. I see this now in some patients who have been with me for a while.

I recently had a family terminate my services. It was a Saturday night at 9:30 PM and I was texted with a complaint of a child who was six years old:

> Mom: "This is Y's throat tonight. I noticed she felt warm tonight with red cheeks, so I checked her throat. It's bright red with bumps on each side of her tonsils."

With it came two pictures of the throat. I looked at the pics and said:

> Me: "Sorry she has been sick. Doesn't look like strep though. I would get her some lozenges and give her some ibuprofen and let's see how she does tomorrow. If it's still bad you can take it to the urgent care, and they can test her."

> Mom: "What does it look like?"

> Me: "A throat without strep. You can never be sure though and so she may want to be tested tomorrow but unless she has a severe sore throat and a fever than I doubt it is strep."

Within minutes I received this from her husband:

> Father: "Please accept this message as our termination of your services. We obviously are not the first to receive curt responses from you as I noticed you referenced it in one of your last emails as you gently raise fees. Z never asked you about strep in her text and if we have to go to urgent care then why are we paying you?"

I have no ill will towards this family. Ok, maybe a little. This is, however, a battle that will continually plague us as we give great services. They get used to it. The above texts came in and I answered them immediately. In retrospect, I probably could have done a better job in my responses, but it is hard to be very eloquent with texting. It was the tone they read into. I talk about that soon in another chapter. Forget the fact that I as soon as I received the information, I evaluated it, and the pics as well, and then gave my professional opinion. I had seen this family for years and did, what I thought, was a great job to meet their needs, which were often excessive. That being said, there is no way they could get this type of service anywhere else. But it didn't matter. Oh, and it was awesome that the father gave me a dig in about my curt responses. There is nothing more hurtful than admitting to your patients you are working on being better only to have them throw it in your face.

Sorry. Back to that lesson later.

Let's look at it another way. The now infamous comedian Louis CK did this bit. Hate him or love him, he is right on target for direct primary care:

> "Everything is amazing right now and nobody's happy. Like, in my lifetime the changes in the world have been incredible… Flying is the worst because people come back from flights and they tell you…a horror story… They're like: "It was the worst day of my life. First of all, we didn't board for twenty minutes, and then we get on the plane and they made us sit there on the runway…" Oh really, what happened next? Did you fly through the air incredibly, like a bird? Did you partake in the miracle of human flight you non-contributing zero?! You're flying! It's amazing! Everybody on every plane should just constantly be going: "Oh my God! Wow!" You're flying! You're sitting in a chair, in the sky!"

Patients get used to your service. They are sitting in the chair in the sky flying the DPC plane. They get used to the immediate responses. They get used to the long visits. They get used to the great service. Sometimes it feels that the more you give, the more they get adapted to it and then the more they expect.

And so goes the treadmill of direct primary care. Speaking of treadmills, this term was changed in the 1990s, by Michael Eysenck to what is now called "hedonic treadmill theory". He compares the pursuit of happiness to a person on a treadmill, who has to keep working just to stay in the same place. This is the observed tendency of humans to quickly return to a relatively stable level of happiness despite major positive or negative events or life changes. In other words, patients get "used to" our positive changes to the culture of primary care and then take it for granted. One mistake or one misinterpretation of your tone can lead to patient turnover or churn. The treadmill never stops. You can only slow it down. I showed you above my example of being terminated by a family so that you know it happens to everyone, including me as I am in the midst of writing this book. It's heartbreaking and I still lose sleep over it. All I can do is try to get better. The next chapter will explain how.

Our Hedonistic Adaptation

One last thing. We, as DPC docs also get hedonistic adaptation. Let's not fool ourselves. After years in the system of seeing 25-30 patients as day, we initially get ecstatic about seeing 8 patients a day. Soon, however, we get spoiled even while seeing those few. Patients can start to irk us as we start getting bombarded with emails or texts. Comparing this to the fee-for-service model, it is an absolute dream but because we became adapted to the good life we start complaining. It's just human nature so all you can do it to try and be aware of it. Life, as a direct primary care doctor, is still good. Remember that. And remember that sometimes we just need to stop bitching.

SECTION TWO:
IDEAS

Chapter Seven:
Working on You

That Darn Mirror

Here is a tough question for your ego. Are you ready? Okay, here goes. Are your patients leaving because of you? Some are because every doctor has a few patients that don't like her. That's called life. But is it possible that you are getting more than your fair share? Listen, you cannot change the person you are, and I am not asking anybody to do that. And I don't want you to take this too personally, though you may. All I want you to do is tweak some of the easier things in order to stop the leakage from your practice.

Most of the following is just about awareness. That is how you get better. Pay attention to what you are doing. You need to try to be present and observe whether there is a need to make some changes. No, I don't want you to dye your hair or get a nose job. But if anyone needed that then I it would be me. But I digress. In my experience, in meeting hundreds and hundreds of DPC docs, it seems to me that you don't need to fix much. They have all been altruistic physicians wanting to help others. I am sure you are the same. So, all you may want to do it is smooth out some of the rough edges. Read the following and just think about it. Don't overthink it and get depressed. You may want to ask your most trusted staff or significant other if there is something here you can work on. Then I would have you just try a few things, even it is just for your professional life, and not anywhere else.

Walk Your Talk

This is going to seem weird, but you do need to be a role model for your patients. This is important. Like it or not, your patients look up to you. You make recommendations for their health all the time and you do this from a position of authority. Therefore, you have to walk your talk. I am not preaching from the mountaintop here because I am right there with you struggling with this. I think I do a pretty good job working on it but in no way am I perfect. So, if you're not doing the things you recommend (diet, exercise, etc.) then your patients will notice. They will lose faith in you. They will lose trust in you. And then they will leave you.

It has been known that doctors who smoke are less likely to talk to their patients about quitting smoking. Granted, this is an older study, and since few doctors smoke now it may not seem relevant, but it is. Let's talk about diet. Listen, if you're overweight and not doing the things you recommend then your patients know it. I am not here to tell you about which diet you should recommend. I am not going to tell you what exercise program is best. I think we both can agree that these things are important, right? So, whatever you conclude then it is best just make sure you're doing it.

How about other things you recommend but don't do? Do you see your own doctor regularly? Do you get your labs regularly? Your patients will ask about this. When you are pointing out their high cholesterol, they may ask about yours. Just be prepared.

Appearance

In my first book I mentioned something about appearance. It really may seem trivial but it's not. You want your patients to see you as that trusted authority. Maybe it's scrubs for you and a white coat. I am not here to tell you what to wear but I do recommend you look professional. For most of you this is going to sound ridiculous but make sure you:

- Shave (men)
- Brush your teeth
- Groom well
- Get new clothes now and then
- Get a haircut regularly

You get the point and you may think I am an idiot for pointing this out. Fine, but I have seen my fair share of doctors with:

- Stained or poorly fitting clothes
- Unshaven
- Massive amount of hair coming out of ears
- Broken and taped glasses
- Bad body odor
- Food in their beard or mustache

Maybe this section wasn't for you. Great. Or maybe it was? Reassess. And then send me a picture.

Actions and Behavior

Now let's take a look at how you treat people. I am sure you are a good doctor and a good person. I am not trying to nitpick here. In fact, this part is MOSTLY for me! I have a ton of trouble with this.

Hopefully you are not doing the really stupid things that get doctors in trouble, right? You know, like telling off-color jokes, saying inappropriate things, or acting unprofessionally? I don't care if you are a wild and crazy guy, in today's atmosphere you need to tone it down.

I have a letter here from Patch Adams, MD. Remember the movie? Patch and I communicated a few times years ago. He used to read my humorous publication, Placebo Journal, and loved it. Since your only reference of Patch may be the film, I want to tell you right here and now that there is NO WAY you can be as spontaneous and crazy as Robin Williams was when he portrayed him. Those days are gone. This does not mean you cannot smile. This does not mean you cannot laugh. This does not mean you cannot ask about your patients' hobbies and jobs and converse about it. This does not mean you cannot talk about sports. In fact, you may interact with your patients more with body language than with anything else.

Psychologist Albert Mehrabian created the 7%-38%-55% rule, which states that three elements can persuade someone to like or hate us or....leave our practice. As crazy as this may seem, words only make up 7% of the message. The tone of voice is 38% and that is crucial especially when interpreted wrongly (see my email chapter). Body language, amazingly enough, is 55%.

Let's talk a little about body language. Much of what we do we are not even conscious we are doing. What's worse is that we judge others' body subconsciously as well. This means you may not even say a word and people can hate or love you. It's not fair but life doesn't care. So, how do you make sure you are not doing things that put people off? Well, you can ask others. You can videotape yourself. There are courses just in this area. I don't have all the answers for you. What I can share you with are the basics and they are:

- Try not to slouch when listening or talking to patients.
- Try not to cross or open your legs in some weird ways.
- Sit up straight in the chair.
- Be careful you are not doing weird fidgeting things. One of my ex-medical partners used to pull at his cheek and make

squishy noises while people talked. I'm not kidding. And a patient complained.

- Be careful how you touch someone and always have a chaperone for full exams of the opposite sex (if not for everyone).

- Work on your posture. Stand tall and straight. It not only makes you feel better but it also projects confidence to your patients.

- Have a comfortable distance from people. Don't be a close talker.

- Make eye contact. This is the biggest complaint about doctors in the FFS model, especially in the EHR era.

- Be careful where you put your arms or hands. When you cross arms, for example, it comes off that you are bothered by the patient.

- Have a firm handshake. If you shake someone's hand like a wet fish then they think of you as weak. I used to wrestle all the way through college and we all thought a weak handshake was a tell-tale sign of an easy match.

- Be genuinely interested in others and your body language will show it.

- Slow down. Slow down your speech. Don't interrupt. Slow down the visit.

- Be personable. Yes, you have to be intentional here. Keep the patient's personal information in the chart and ask about it.

- Hugging all your patients, unfortunately, is a no go anymore. Be very, very careful with this.

Is It Your Staff?

Everything I wrote above applies to your staff as well. I've been very lucky in that I have a great assistant, who is awesome, as well as a great practice manager, who is my wife. If you're going to evaluate what turns patients off about yourself then you also want to evaluate what your staff is doing. Don't ignore this. Hopefully some of the data you analyzed, as well as feedback you have gotten, will show this. Of course, you want to see if you can train them better but sometimes there is nothing you can do. You are the owner, and this is your practice and your lifeblood so don't be hesitant to make tough decisions and take action here. Evaluate, change or train them, or fire them if it can't be done. Now if your spouse is your practice manager then be very careful with this. This can affect your marriage so…..hold on….my wife is coming…need to stop here.

I'm back. Wow, that was a close one.

Okay, that was an uncomfortable chapter. Sorry. Oh, and I still fail often with this so don't look to me as someone who is perfect. But I am working on it and while researching this section I realized I can be so much better. Maybe you can be as well?

Chapter Eight:
The Traps of Email and Texting

I know what you are saying, "This guy is going tell me how to answer an email or text?" The answer is yes! After evaluating some of the most ridiculous reasons people have left my practice, I would have to say making mistakes using email or text have been one of the most common. But is it possible they weren't so ridiculous after all? Patients are paying for a service and they want everything from that service to be done in a top-notch way. If you leave any wiggle room while emailing or texting where they can infer inappropriate tone, then you must assume that they will.

In direct primary care, use of technology has been an awesome way to give great service to patients without having them unnecessarily come in to be seen. It saves on visits, for both the patient and you, while still giving great care. Though this is a godsend in many ways it can definitely be burdensome and wear the practitioner down. This is where problems start to happen. If done correctly, you really can save yourself a lot of unnecessary visits as well as do a great job for your patients. If done poorly, you can lose patients who read into anything you say especially if you don't know the patient or if they are someone who dissects every word that you write or text. This is not to denigrate them in anyway. This is just human nature.

One of the things that has been troubling to me in my own practice has been the amount of access, via email, patients have had. Even though it is a selling point to my practice, it has tended to sour me when I get barraged with emails that really tend to be minimal or non-urgent. Since I have a personality that wants to get things done immediately, I tended to answer these emails as quickly as I got them. Though that takes the pressure off me and made me feel better, it still caused me problems. I would answer quickly feeling that it would make the patient feel responded to but, because I did not pay attention to how I answered the emails, they often would take some of my answers the wrong way even though they were not intended to be that way.

Let me give you some real examples where I lost, or almost lost, a few patients:

EXAMPLE ONE:

> *Elderly patient's daughter: Dr. Farrago can you send an order to PT for X to be evaluated for strengthening her legs? She likes Y at PT and feels like some PT will help her. They have appts this week if they can get the order. Medicare will not cover without a doctor's order. Thank you.*
>
> *ME: She needs a new diagnosis for rehab. What would that be?*
>
> *Daughter: What about gait abnormality?*
>
> *ME: Is this new? We just can't ask for PT anytime we want?*

Daughter: Yes, I guess this is new. We have been after her to see you about the weakness in her legs and hands, but you know mom. Now that she is coming to Y, she thought that maybe she could be evaluated and do some PT if it would help. Do you need to see her?

ME: Yes, there has to be an exam by me first. Maybe next week or the week after if we have time.

The patient was relayed these messages in real time and was upset at my responses and decided to leave the practice. I still do not know exactly which of my answers bothered her, but I assumed it was the initial rejection and the timeframe to get in.

EXAMPLE TWO:

PATIENT: Hi, Do you have a basic questionnaire for assessing a two year old for autism? I think X is fine, but I've observed some quirky tendencies- not consistent. Definitely not like Y, but at the same time I missed some things with Y that I questioned in my head then he would meet his development milestones and I wouldn't think about it for a while again. Anyway, Y has mild, high functioning autism and I would like peace of mind that I'm not missing anything on X. It's been bugging me for a few weeks so if you have a screening assessment that you use, can you forward it to me please. Thanks! Z

ME: I do not have one. Sorry. Dr. F

PATIENT: I remember at our last pediatrician's office they gave one for Y almost like a prescreening. I don't know how many young pediatric patients you see, but I think it would be beneficial for your practice and your families with young children to offer some kind of questionnaire. He isn't in preschool this year. He will go next year.

ME: Here is the evidence which is very inconclusive on whether screening should be done. When parents have a child they are concerned about then we further pursue a more official evaluation via a referral. A large amount of this practice is pediatric, btw: https://www.uspreventiveservicestaskforce.org/Announcements/News/Item/final-recommendation-statement-screening-for-autism-spectrum-disorder-in-young-children

PATIENT: Thanks for the info. I appreciate this more than your first response.

ME: At every physical I still ask developmental questions based on age to see if there is a concern. Unfortunately, I try to answer patients emails as fast as I get them and sometimes it's between seeing other patients. They are not always as lengthy as people like, but I do the best I can.

PATIENT: Sounds good! Thank you for the insight and for the clarification. Most times I appreciate the short responses, but in this case the education/info was greatly appreciated! I know we aren't mind readers. We really appreciate you and your office!

ME: Totally understand. You're welcome. Sorry for any confusion.

This is an example of where my initial answer was way too short for a very complicated and worrisome issue to a parent. I cringe reading it now. I backtracked later when I saw what I did, and it helped. It could have been prevented. This family stayed with me.

EXAMPLE THREE:

After a recent round of almost a dozen emails with rapid answers by me to questions about medication use, the patient responded with this:

"Have I done something to personally offend you? Because you seemed quite curt in your last couple emails to me, as well."

This patient and his spouse eventually left the practice. After fully reviewing the chart I found that my emails were becoming shorter and shorter and did come off curt. He was correct. I'm not sure if I could've done many things differently as I had answered so many of his emails which were sometimes 6 to 10 paragraphs long with the best effort that I thought I could. It just goes to show you that sometimes you can only do so much and if people see a change in your responses, they will tend to read into it. None of my responses were negative but they seemed to have gotten shorter in length. This gentleman took offense and left because of this.

These examples are only a few of the many over my years in direct primary care. You have to remember that we are different than regular fee-for-service offices. Those offices do not truly answer their emails. Many times, they are totally ignored. Other times, nurses are basically relaying the answers from their physicians. In the world of metrics, these offices only need to answer a certain small percentage to get bonused by insurers. We live in a different world. Our world is to go beyond the normal expectations and create an experience that patients can brag about to their friends. Sometimes this can border on ridiculous. I once had a patient text me with a question just to prove to a friend that his doctor was at his fingertips. He was out at a bar and asked about something meaningless. I knew it when I saw it and it was bothersome. It didn't matter to him that I felt like I was being pimped out. These situations are not the norm, but it just goes to show you what the mindset is of some patients paying a monthly service. This is an extreme example and something we really don't have to get into here. More importantly, you have to ignore these extremes and deal with the most common emails and texts that come your way. You cannot let these outliers affect how you deal with everyone else. Other patients don't know you been handling ridiculous text or emails from others. All they know about is what they are telling you in their own emails or texts. And that is ALL they care about.

One way I decided to fix the barrage of communications I was getting was to batch my emails. I needed to explain to patients why I was doing this in order to not make them feel they weren't being heard. This plan helped me as long as I did truly batch these emails, which is still a problem for me today, but I try. What I did was use an automatic vacation response on my email that every patient received. That way they understood why there was a delay in my response. Here are two examples, one by me and one by another DPC doctor (Dr. Allison Edwards), who's doing the same thing.

Thanks for your email. I will get back to you with an answer bu*t in order to give my full attention to your question I will be batching all my emails to a few isolated times throughout the day. I find this allows me to answer your question more fully and respectfully without coming off curt or rude due to its brevity. Because of this change I cannot give you an exact time I will get back to you, but I guarantee it will be within 24 hours. If you feel your question is more urgent, then leave the word URGENT in the subject line and then text me at XXX with "Urgent: see email". Always know that you can call me at the same number if there is an emergency. In fact, if I don't answer your urgent text in a timely manner then you will have to call me.*

I am sorry if this is an inconvenience for you. I am making this change to see if I can be a better doctor and in order to do that, I need to concentrate on the patients I see during the day while isolating other times to concentrate on the emails I receive. Thank you for being understanding.

Sincerely,

Douglas Farrago MD

Thanks for emailing!

In an effort to cut down on distractions throughout the day, my emails will only arrive in my inbox weekdays at 8:30am, 12:00pm, and 3:30pm. This means I may not see your email immediately! If you have something that needs to be addressed more urgently and the clinic is open, please call the clinic at X.

If there is an urgent matter that cannot wait until I'm back in the office, please reach out by phone.

Thanks!

Dr. Edwards

As you can see, this allows me and Dr. Edwards to have breathing room and more time to get back to somebody. The goal is then to spend time on that email and answer in an appropriate way so that patients can be happy with the response. If things are urgent, they can text me and I will then spend more time on that email immediately. Dr. Edwards allows them to call so things are dealt with urgently. This leaves little room for mistakes to happen even though it's still possible.

Now let's get to the meat of this section. How do you get better? Well, the answer isn't easy, but it can be done. If you ignore this, however, it can set you back and you will lose patients who you don't need to lose. It is always great to get new patients into your practice, but that is even harder work than you think. The better plan is make sure you keep the patients you have, especially the good ones, happy. That's the crux of this book but this section explains how something as simple as how you answer your texts or emails can stop you from falling into an easy trap that is hard to climb out of.

In his book, *Pre-suasion*, Robert Cialdini Ph.D., explains how to prepare people to be receptive to a message before they experience it. He even quotes Sun Tzu from the book *The Art of War* where he says, "Every battle is won before it is fought". This is all true as it relates to dealing with patients, especially via email and texts. You do NOT want to battle with patients. You want to win before you even start. Cialdini illustrates how the artful diversion of attention leads to successful pre-suasion and gets your patient primed and ready to say, "yes" instead of them arguing with you about your response or worse, taking what you said the wrong way and later quitting. That is what was happening to me. Cialdini's major point is this: "Before introducing a message, arrange to make your audience sympathetic to it". In other words, what we present first, changes the way people experience what we present to them next.

Does this sound crazy to you? It did to me. Cialdini's book is mostly about marketing but it relates directly to how we communicate to patients electronically. Why? In an article by David Swink, in Psychology today, (https://www.psychologytoday.com/us/blog/threat-management/201311/dont-type-me-email-and-emotions) he warns of the following:

- Just because you write in a certain way doesn't mean it's received the same way. Compose your email recognizing that the receiver may not be in the same mood or emotional state as you. Try to imagine how the person receiving the email could interpret it.

- When we read an email, we attempt to read intention and tone into the words. If the message is ambiguous, many people will automatically read the most negative emotions and intentions into it.

- If you think there is room for misinterpretation of your message, take the time to craft the email to make sure your message is more likely to be received with your true intention. This might make the email longer.

- Most people know by now that typing in ALL CAPS is the same as screaming at someone.

- Don't overuse punctuation!!!!

- If you are not sure about the tone of an email you are sending, have someone else read it and give you feedback before you send it. If no one else is available for a tone check, park the email in your draft folder and come back and re-read it a couple of hours later before sending it.

- Most importantly, know when to pick up the phone or meet face-to-face to discuss an issue.

Hopefully this now makes sense to you. So how do we fix this? It's simple. You need to always answer your emails or texts with some phrase or phrases that makes your audience or patients sympathetic to what you are going to say next. Let's not get too crazy here. Basically, what I'm saying is you need to start with empathy, throw some empathy in the middle section and then end with empathy. That's it. Does that sound too hard? Well, sometimes it is if you are responding to one of those ridiculous questions from a patient. For example, "Hey, doc, why does my gas smell bad?". As much as you want to shoot back with something rude and offensive, don't. The answer is not to get caught up in what the patient is saying or who the patient is. You need to make this automatic so that your emotions do not get involved. The way to do this is as easy as using the examples I give below. And use them without thinking about it. You can even make a game out of it and just spin the wheel and pick any of the responses below. That will save you so much heartache in the end, I can't even tell you. It has worked for me with great success. In fact, patients are much more appreciative. This may be my best lesson in this whole book. One more thing, this is not a trick. You are a great doctor who is empathetic. You are feeling these things in your heart and saying them in your head. You just aren't writing them, probably due to time. In other words, you are not being disingenuous by using my tips below.

Empathetic email beginnings:

- Happy to help (This is the Josh Umbehr, MD special).
- Sorry to hear that.
- This must be hard for you.
- That's a great question.
- I'm sorry you are going through this.
- Great question, let me find out for you.
- I'm sorry that this happened.

- That must be hard.
- That would frustrate me too.
- I would be asking the same questions as you are.
- If I'm understanding you correctly...
- So what you're saying is...
- That sounds really challenging.
- I can see how that would be difficult.
- Let me help you with that.
- What I'm hearing is that you are feeling _____. Is that right?
- I want to make sure I understand...

Empathetic email middle content:

- You can consider X.
- You might find X helpful
- You are totally right.
- I would come to the same conclusion.
- I would think the same thing but...
- I think you'll find it's much easier if you do X.

Empathetic email endings:

a. Is there anything else that I can help you with today?
b. I wish I could make it better but...
c. I hope this was helpful for you.
d. Please keep me updated on how things go.
e. Is there anything else you want to share?
f. Always know that I'm in your corner.
g. I'm happy to listen anytime.
h. I'm here for you if you need anything else.

I highly recommend you keep adding and changing the above, so it sounds like your voice. I also recommend you rotate these often so as not to give what sounds like a "canned" response. In other words, if people keep seeing the same line they may become a little suspicious.

To summarize, people will read your emails in many different ways. It all depends on their mood, how sick they are, and their overall disposition or personality. You have to always be aware of this and how it affects your responses. I do recommend you batch your emails so you don't get caught answering them in what seems to be rude or curt manner. (See my last chapter and the guy who hammered me for this). I recommend you use my empathetic responses both at the beginning, the middle, and the end of each email. If you can do this with texts then great, but that is really hard. Texting tends to be very short by nature. I recommend you tell them to resend their question, if it isn't simple, to you via email. You also don't always have to answer each email immediately and, in fact, you don't want to because that may get you in trouble like it did me. Try to train your patients to understand that emails will be answered when you can give them the time needed for an appropriate response and then when you do answer those emails use my recommendations above.

Chapter Nine:
Showing That You Care

Dammit, Jim, I'm a doctor, not a counselor. Yes, I've heard it before. You are a physician who prides herself in doing your job and getting things done. Great. I am here to tell that this may not be enough. I'm actually asking you to show that you care. Why? Here's the thing. I have no idea who you are, but I have an idea of where you've been and that place could NOT give a crap if you cared about your patients or not. You just needed to see lots of patients and bill them hard. The world of direct primary care is the exact opposite. You are giving patients a different level of service and your monthly paying members need to see a difference in their doctor. Some of you, however, are still stuck in that fee-for-service model where you still are a robodoc moving from room to room, patient to patient. That's not going to work anymore and if you can't change then this really isn't for you. You need do tear down the walls built by the FFS system and begin anew. "Dr. Gorbachev tear down those walls"!

It's been said that patients don't care how much you know until they know how much you care. I am not sure where that's from, but I do think it's right on the money and the essence of this whole chapter. What I'm going to share with you is what I have found to be helpful to show patients that you ACTUALLY care about them. There is one caveat, however, you must know. Even if you truly care, in your heart, about your patients but they don't perceive this then it doesn't matter. I'm not saying it's fair, but I am saying it's a reality. In fact, the reverse is true. Those who don't care as much as you can still look better and retain patients longer because they are doing the following things. Here are ways that you can show you care so they do perceive it and stay longer.

Following Up

I mention this in my first book, but I need to reiterate how important this is. Try to go back into your last week's schedule and just pick three or four people you can check on. Then send them emails and see how they were doing after you saw them. Some common ones for me are infections, depression or an injury. Maybe it is checking on how their kid is doing? Try not to ask the same people over and over. I also do this on Monday mornings only. Nothing shows you "care" more than asking how someone has been doing after they saw you. Usually, they are so impressed by this that you may never lose them as patients. As I write this, I just got this response, "Thanks for checking in. That is AWESOME!!" and this, "Thank you so much for following up. It really means a lot.

Read Up

Nothing makes you look dumber then when a patient says, "Remember, I told you that last month?" Yet, it still happens to me occasionally. It used to happen to me all the time in the FFS model. My former partner was notorious for this. In fact, I remember him complaining about one patient whose story kept changing over and over again. He whined that she seemed to forget a lot of things he would tell her. That's when our other medical partner said to him,

"You know she is a twin and you have both sisters, right?". His response was, "What?" Yeah, he didn't know he was seeing two different patients.

There are no more excuses anymore in DPC, but even I still blow it now and then. I hate when I fall into any trap where I look like an idiot. Not reading up and remembering things about a patient is an avoidable one. It just takes about five minutes to look at what your last note said, and to scan the personal section. Then you won't be caught off guard. Even better, you will look so much better in the patient's eyes. Dare I say you're also doing a better job? It really impresses

patients when you do the simplest thing like remembering what happened during their past visits. Once again it shows you care, and it blows away what other doctors are doing in the fee-for-service model.

Personal Section of the EMR

I don't know what EMR you use but Atlas MD has a great "Personal Notes" section in their EMR where I keep it updated about their jobs, hobbies, and other things to remember them by. For kids, I ask about their pets, their favorite movie, their favorite books, etc. I do try to look at this and bring things up each year. Not in a superficial manner. I try to be genuinely interested. Listen, DPC is a lonely sport, especially if you have no partners. Your patients can replace some of the social interactions you lose by working alone. And you will be surprised how much you can learn. It also helps you to never forget about the patient. Also, it may open your eyes to their business models and may help in networking. I have gotten companies to join because of this.

Find Out Why They Didn't Show

The term "no show" has a definite reaction for physicians. When I was in residency, I loved it because it gave me some breathing room. I used to do a "no show" dance before my clinic started, kind of like a shaman dancing for rain. When I was early in my fee-for-service career and had a guaranteed income, I also loved it and did the same dance. When I started really working on a eat-what-you-kill revenue model, in a hospital-employed practice, I did a 180 degree turn and started getting upset when they didn't show up. Hell, I was losing money! In my last year of being employed and knowing that I was leaving, I went back to a guaranteed contract and again was doing the "no-show" dance each morning, hoping patients wouldn't show up. I guess my point is that I have been all over the place with this issue.

You would think that in direct primary care having a no-show would be cool because you're still getting paid. Unfortunately, it's actually a problem if people aren't showing up on your schedule. I would highly recommend that you email these people personally. Don't use staff. Ask them what happened and how you can get them back in. People who no-show are wasting appointments for others. Even worse, they could be valuing their membership less, which means they may soon quit. You need to find out and address it.

Related to this, another thing we're doing is going back using the Atlas.MD EMR to see when patients were last seen. If it has been over a year, then I am personally emailing them to see if we can get them in for a physical.

All this shows that you care. You care that they pay attention to their health. It shows them you don't want to just take money from them. That means a lot.

The Easy Ones

Send out condolence cards when a patient has a death in the family. You can get nice condolence cards cheap on Amazon. If you want to write it yourself, great. For me, my handwriting is an issue. Make sure you at least sign it. If you can leave a little note, then even better.

Try to mention birthdays when patients are in for their visits. This is rare for adults but we normally schedule kids' physicals around their birthdays. Make sure you bring it up and ask what presents they got. This means a lot to the kids and the parents. For the adults, Atlas MD has an automatic birthday email that gets sent out. Ours looks like this:

> Happy birthday [patient's first name]!
>
> Debbie, Christine and I wish you a day filled with all your favorite things. We thank you for being a part of Forest Direct Primary Care.
>
> Sincerely,
>
> Douglas Farrago MD

You can get other cards on Amazon as well that say "congratulations" on them. Use these for graduations or promotions if you find out about them. These little things add up. You can do the same for some simple accomplishments such as losing weight or as big as completing a marathon.

We also have a set of "thank you" cards for any patient that referred someone else to come see us. We do that for every referral, no matter if the patient joins or not. We always ask patients who come visit us how they heard about us. This tips us off about who referred them. Those patients love that we do this.

Lastly, think about sending out anniversary emails or handwritten notes. It can be a thank you for staying with you for one, two, three years and so on. People love feeling appreciated.

People want to feel noticed and feel good about themselves. Sending out personal notes or cards is a simple way we can insert ourselves into their lives. All it takes is having a staff person and/or yourself taking the extra two minutes to write these cards out. Do not underestimate how much this helps you keep patients.

10

Chapter Ten:
Create A Community Around
Your Practice

I think one of the best things we have done in our practice is to make it feel like one big family. I cannot take credit for that. My wife, Debbie, who is my practice manager, comes in the mornings and is always social with patients. She talks to them if they have to wait. She will play Old Maid with their kids. And she is always nice and smiling. Christine, my assistant and phlebotomist, has been with us from the beginning. Patients love her because she knows them all and is extremely caring, respectful and kind to them.

I believe I have added some to this "family" feeling here but it would not be enough without these two people. But that is ok. My patients know it is a team here and they feel part of that team. They know pretty soon that they are getting access to something rare that others don't get. They know that they feel special in the office and are treated really well. They also know we are filled and that they are part of a select group looking out versus looking in. It is behind the velvet rope where patients feel a certain sense of status being in my practice. That status is not costly. That status can be thought of as a community.

Do you ever wonder why CrossFit is successful? It's not only because they have a good product that people like. The bigger part may just be their sense of community. Clients seem to know each other and enjoy being together. The trainers are Crossfitters and like what they do and show it by being helpful. Everyone there is like-minded in their attitudes toward fitness, and they feel special to be a part of the group. I am jealous as I can't do CrossFit due to my total knee replacement, but I know enough people who do that and I wish I could participate. I want to get past the CrossFit velvet rope. It sucks being old.

Direct primary care is not the same as CrossFit. I get that. Patients never see each other so they don't really know each other. We are at a disadvantage with that because we never have patients sitting around waiting to be seen. That being said, I can't tell you how many times people get surprised to discover that their friend or co-worker is coming to see me if they happen to run into each other in the office. It never gets old seeing them brag to each other about us. So how can DPC create that CrossFit community without patients knowing each other? The following is what I came up with.

Lectures

Lectures work pretty well because patients can come together and talk before and after I speak. Patients can then meet each other. It's actually very nice to see them mingle and feel part of our DPC community. This really works if you do it exclusively for patients only. I recommend you say no when people ask to bring a friend or, if you want to build your practice, allow them only ONE guest. This creates FOMO for those patients' friends who hear you speak and want to be part of the practice and be your patient. I mention this more in a later chapter.

Online

You can create a FB group that is private and only for confirmed patients. You just need to clearly define what you can say publicly due to HIPAA. You would put a disclaimer in the FB page. You would remove any patients that leave your practice and keep adding new ones on. You have to be the administrator and sometimes mediate disagreements, but it is still worth it. Topics to discuss could be articles you highlight in your newsletter or just new studies coming out. You can also highlight things going on in your practice. You can also spotlight and thank patients here. Patients may help one another with some questions. All this may provide your patients with a platform to engage with other patients. They can also give you great feedback. You can analyze their conversations so that it may help you tweak your office and even slightly change the way you practice medicine. It will also help create lasting relationships with patients; the purpose of this book. I know this is more work for you so make sure you have the time to participate. It is another good example of the velvet rope area that patients may really like taking part in.

You can do the same thing with YouTube and make your videos private for only your patients.

Sponsor An Event

You can sponsor an event like a race or for a charity and be there when it occurs. We do this for a few different events and charities. This also lends itself to community. Obviously, you are doing this for the right reasons but the collateral effect is people coming together in a family atmosphere.

Chapter Eleven:
Don't Let Them Forget The Value of Your Services

One of the biggest frustrations for me as a DPC doc is that I feel like I'm giving tremendous value to patients and yet I've heard some patients, upon leaving, feel they may not have received their money's worth. Others don't say anything and yet I see then transferring to a regular fee-for-service model office. This happens even though I have done so many procedures on them that were complimentary in our practice. Were they using us to get these extras done? Maybe. More likely is that they may not understand the cost of things. This is typical of the medical system which hides the cost of everything and has trained patients to be ignorant of cost. That's why they use a technique to bill a patient much later on, so the patient almost forgets about what was done. I'm not sure people would want to pay $178 for some cryotherapy if any of that was the cost coming out of their pocket right then and there. This is why I make a habit of emailing them later with the actual cost of their services. I was tipped off about this when I saw a receipt from Kohl's department store which told me how much money I was saving. I felt great about it and thought maybe my patients would as well.

Presently, I send out an email after seeing a patient for a visit that includes any procedure. The email "nicely" shows how much they would have paid somewhere else. Here is my template. Feel free to steal it.

> It was good to see you today. We love treating patients and LOVE saving them money! In today's visit you had _____ which would normally* cost $_____ at other offices. Here it just comes with your membership. As always, thank you for being part of Forest Direct Primary Care.
>
> Sincerely,
>
> Dr. Farrago
>
> *source:https://www.fairhealthconsumer.org

I also keep a list of prices for my most common procedures from that reference above so it is always handy.

List of prices: https://www.fairhealthconsumer.org

1. Abscess: $215
2. Level three established office visit (99213): $130
3. Level four established office visit (99214): $200
4. Punch or shave biopsy: $166
5. Cryotherapy: $178 (up to 14)
6. Mole removal: $275

    a. Intermediate layer closure: $462

7. Ear wax:

    a. One - $103 add $28 with washing

    b. Two - $206, add $56 with washing

8. EKG: $52

9. Lac repair

    a. Less than 2.5 cm

        i. $272

       ii. ADD $752 if done in hospital

10. OMT – 5 to 6 levels $98

    a. 6-7 is $118

You can, and should, make your own list and update it. I have never had a negative comment about this email. I have also read other experts recommending this as well. If you don't do this then you run the risk of patients taking some of your work for granted and that is not fair to you. Out of sight, out of mind.

In my office, I do these emails personally so that they know it is from me as the doctor. I guess the staff could send them out, but it is just as easy to have this template as a macro on my EMR. I usually send them out at the end of the day and include both the office visit fee and the procedure in the email. We save more money on labs for patients and that could be another reminder that could be sent. I have not done this because I think the amount of time would be prohibitive since we do a lot of labs. But it could be done and would not only be appropriate but may help you even more to keep patients. Lastly, some patients share these "savings" emails with friends and family members, which is free marketing for you.

Chapter Twelve:
Are They Using You Enough?

This is a tough chapter to understand because, as I told you before, there are certain patients who you don't want to overuse you. There is a happy balance of who you want to give your energy to. You have to be diligent here and learn not to cater to the very small percentage that are abusing you. I know that's a very strong word to use, but there are certain patients that you need to train not to overuse you. In my experience, I find those people are the first to leave you anyway. The Pareto principle applies here, but I think it is more 5% abusive and 95% that you need to work on using you enough.

Training

All great comedians and magicians owe much of their success less to their material and more to the setup. The same goes for you. If you don't work on expectations and education by teaching or training patients about how the system works, then eventually it will get you in trouble.

In this book I already talked about emails and your responses and the time you will get back to people. You are going to have to learn to set boundaries for some people detailing your availability and how quickly you'll respond to them. You are not their personal butler. You are a caring physician who knows how to triage certain issues and you will get them as soon as possible, especially when things are not emergencies.

For some people you actually have to hold back the reigns on when you get them in and when you answer their emails and texts. This is a for a very small minority of your patients who don't understand that they are not your only patients. I know this can come off negatively but it's extremely important to know when running your practice. You have to train your patients so that expectations of your service can still be high yet reasonable. For example, in my practice I send a lot of emails and newsletters about common colds. I state that I don't need to see them if there is nothing I can do and I don't want to expose anyone else to their illness, which is untreatable and will go away on its own. I have some standard responses for basic viral illnesses that hopefully keeps them happy and educated but doesn't waste an office visit in my schedule. This way patients feel listened to while not being a burden to my day or to other patients. What I mean by that is no one patient is more important than another.

I cannot make everyone happy, however. I had someone recently demand to be seen first thing in the morning for a sore throat. She texted me urgently at 7 AM. I heard her complaint and felt it was really minor. I nicely explained to her that I cannot cancel other patients' appointments just for her and that a sore throat is probably viral. I told this patient I will get her in as soon as I can if she feels she needs to be seen. I teased out that there was no fever, that her symptoms had just started and that it probably needs more time with the use of lozenges and ibuprofen. And yet she still demanded to be seen that morning. This is a red flag. I did see her later that morning and the strep test was negative, the exam was benign, and as much as I did a dog and pony show to make her happy, it didn't seem to work. Now is that the kind of patient who I need in my practice? Probably not and the truth is this family has been using me over and over again for very small issues that they ALWAYS make urgent. Is that really worth it? Well, since my practice is filled, probably not. All I can do is be honest, open, caring and try to train them better. For them, it has not worked and so I will not be worried if she is still not happy because this is not a practice for her. I will now slow my responses to her and see what happens (see my thoughts on this in an earlier chapter). I don't want to lose my mind trying to make them happy, and I refuse to lose what's left of my overtaxed brain.

This book is more for those people who you are not seeing enough. Those are the ones you have to keep engaged and excited to be part of your direct primary care practice. Why? They say that patient turnover or churn is directly related to use. In other words, people want to get their money's worth. I know physicians who are extremely happy when no one is on their schedule. This, however, can be problematic. If people aren't finding value in your subscription model DPC practice, then they are going to eventually leave. Your competition is not other practices, as I've said before. Those fee-for-service models don't care if people stay with them because they are overwhelmed anyway. For you, your competition is your patient's denial, inertia, laziness, and willpower. What does that mean? If they just "set it and forget it" with their billing when they sign up, then they will eventually cancel their subscriptions. You want to change their behavior so that they are using you appropriately. That means coming regularly for their physicals or following up on certain medical issues. This means getting their labs when they need to be done and, if they cancel or miss appointments, then you follow up and make sure they do come in. This shows you care, which blows their minds. This is very different and disruptive from what they will see in the FFS medical environment. People are not used to that, but it is a positive for your practice. This also makes it a habit for them that they know they are accountable to their physician and medical office and to their own health.

Remember, one of the biggest reasons people stop subscribing to any service is the perception that they are paying for something they are not using. You want them using you. Again, you need to exclude the ones who are "challenging" you. These are the abusers and the jumpers. There is a sweet spot of use and you just know when someone is over that limit. They say the stickiest subscription businesses make it their mission to insert themselves into the daily lives of their customers. They are "stickin' or they are quittin". So how can you do that?

What I am going to show you are techniques that keep them interested and keep their attention while not overtaxing you as the doctor. It includes ways that integrate your practice into their daily lives and insert your service into their routines without being a nuisance.

Chapter Thirteen:
Using Social Media

In my first book I talked about how to use social media, especially Facebook, in marketing your practice. As I said, part of slowing the churn rate is to actually market to your own patients. What does that mean? Patients are having a ton of problems navigating the healthcare system. This could be due to cost or access or both. This is the conversation going on in their heads and you want to be involved with it.

I still post regularly on Facebook even though my practice is filled. I do that to keep my brand alive as well as constantly reminding others that we are still around. You would be amazed at how many potential patients are trolling you for years. I still get people joining my practice who have followed me since the first article came out in the paper five years ago who then followed me on Facebook. Remember, people are bombarded by posts all the time. It's like throwing a small twig into a massive waterfall. In the old days it may take only a few of these touch points to finally get them to come in. Now it may take years and hundreds, if not thousands, of posts. That may be ridiculous, but it is reality.

Social media also enables my patients to get involved in these posts by adding their own comments to them. When I give opinions about certain subjects, whether it's healthcare or even medical issues, they tend to get involved. This reinforces to them why they are staying with me. My thoughts, recommendations, commentary and advice are not only beneficial to them when they read it, but they end up spreading it to their friends. There is nothing like hearing someone say, "That's my doctor!". When they brag about you it is tougher for them to leave later on, which slows the churn.

Facebook has changed since I first started. In the beginning they would let all of my followers, who liked my practice, read all of the posts. Facebook has figured out that they want to make more money and they're pushing you to boost these posts. They do this by exposing your posts to only a small percentage of your followers. Ugh. There is no way around it and though it's unfair, you still have to play the game. I probably post $50 to $100 worth every month which now is mostly my only form of marketing. It's still gets new patients but like I said, it reinforces what patients like about us and it makes them feel part of the community.

What and How Often?

I get it. You don't have time to be a social media guru. You don't want to keep having to create new content. This gets more ingrained in your head as your practice is almost filled or fully filled. But remember, you're trying to market to your own people and many of them are on Facebook following you. Don't ignore this. You need to post regularly, which I believe should be at least once or twice a week. You don't even have to push for people to join your practice on each post. Your job is really just to educate people, which shows you are on their side as well as establishing you as authoritative figure or expert. And you are! You're a doctor! Think of the other idiots putting absolute crap out there. You are doing a service by drowning them out. Sometimes I just post about how we just saved a patient a lot of money with labs. I may state that I just did a thyroid screening test for only $10 versus $110 and picked up someone's hypothyroidism, which would not have been found in a FFS model because of cost. I leave it that and then people want to find out more. Even better is that this reinforces to your own patients why they stay with you.

Be careful not to post right on top of a previous post. Facebook does not like that and will ignore your first post, which wastes your time. You can do a lot of posts at one time and then schedule them out so your stuff isn't on top of itself and diluted. You should also be looking regularly for good articles that come out on topics you want to comment on. This could be medical topics that you have an affinity for or newspaper articles written about other DPC offices. I just co-opt them and explain how proud I am of them for opening up their own practice. I then explain how we do the same service. I highly recommend you sign up with pocket.com, which is free, where you can easily save Internet articles and then go back and use them later.

Video

Whether you like it or not, Facebook prefers video. It's what they're pushing because they like original content that people can be engaged with. I have done videos since the beginning of my practice but never really pushed them early on in Facebook. That has changed. Facebook also loves video that is live, and though I'm still not great at that, it is something I am working on.

But you're squeamish about being on film? Too bad. Times have changed and you have to go along with it. Go ahead and look at other peoples' Facebook videos and you will see how unprofessional they look but are still very effective. You also get confident by looking at these videos and realizing you can do the same thing.

The new smart phones have such good video quality that all you need is to turn it on after you practice a few times. I highly recommend getting a mic that you can plug in to your smart phone, which enables the audio to be of high quality. There's nothing more bothersome than when someone clicks on your video and can't hear you. They will shut it off. You can do this with a Yeti mic or even a lavalier mic.

But what do you talk about? I think content is king and you do need to have a topic that is important. What's interesting is that it is not different than anything else you have been doing by written posts. If it is a topic about the health care system and how direct primary care improves that model, then go ahead and talk about it. Or maybe it's a disease process where you think your office can do a better job than the normal fee-for-service model. Don't make the video too long, be personable and authentic, and then post the sucker. I also recommend boosting these when you can.

People want to put a face to your practice. I know some doctors who even post very personal issues via video (about themselves or their family) and that's fine too if you're open to it. It connects people to you emotionally and again makes you more human, which most doctors have a bad reputation of not being. Put yourself in your patients' shoes. They want someone they can actually talk to and now they're seeing that person talk on a video in the same way they would be spoken to in the office. They now see their doctor as a regular person. Once again, this helps not only in recruiting new patients but it reinforces why your patients like you so much.

Chapter Fourteen:
Miscellaneous Ideas

N ow let's have a little fun. What I have put together is as many ideas that I thought up myself as well as what I have gleaned from other books and articles. I also have some recommendations I have taken liberally from other industries and even other DPC docs. I highly recommend you try as many as you can on a regular basis. You want to be constant and consistent. You can do things over and over again but space them out. Remember, by sometimes surprising and delighting your patients, you are showing them that you are always there and that you care. It may seem overwhelming, but it really isn't, especially if you can get your staff involved. There really isn't any rhyme or reason to the order I give below. I will try to give some explanation for each one.

Have an In-House Pharmacy

We don't do this because it was too much of a pain in my state of Virginia. That is not to say it can't be done and I know another new DPC doc who is trying to pull this off. For other states it is much easier. The extra effort of stocking, dispensing and organizing may well be worth the increased savings for patients. Do NOT underestimate how much those savings will keep your patients from leaving. Not only is this great for slowing the churn but it also great for marketing. Patients will brag and when they do then it is harder for them to leave.

The Gold Card

Right from the beginning I knew the feeling of exclusivity was important to our patients. Even when I wasn't filled, I created a very expensive, as compared to other business cards, Gold Card. On it I put my cell number and email address. We tell them this is for patient's only and it is a direct line to me. They eat it up. It's like they have access to the Bat Signal to call Batman. They feel so special and it is something to brag about to their friends. It's free advertising. Also, anytime someone brags about something that you do for them it psychologically makes it harder for them to leave (and throw out the card).

Get Patients to Review You

I recommend you get patients to give you nice reviews on Facebook, RateMDs, Healthgrades, and Google. Obviously, this will help market your practice as more and more of the public is looking at these rating sites. Unfortunately, when you live by the sword you can die by the sword so be careful to watch these things regularly. I thought I had all bases covered until I saw that I had a one-star rating, with terrible comments, on Yelp and it was from an idiot who drilled us for a ridiculous reason. And it was very hard, if not impossible, to dilute him out. I think Yelp is a scam and so I recommend you research all the issues other businesses are having with them. They refused to put any of my positive comments up that patients have made about us and only leave that one-star rating. In fact, if I was you, I wouldn't even put your information up on Yelp. They are not worth it.

I can say that people who leave nice comments tend not to leave your practice. There is something about patients taking the effort to leave you a review that makes it harder for them to leave your practice. Maybe that's confirmation bias or some other psychological attachment but it works. I recommend you be very careful in asking for reviews. I use emails and my newsletter to garner these, but when they're always positive the rating services will think there is some type of finagling going on. This is because when more than one review is given on a single day, they think you are asking for them, which you are, and then they will eliminate them. That sucks because patients don't want to go through the effort of doing it again. I also find Yelp, for some reasons, to be a tougher in this manner. Yelp only puts on those reviews from reviewers who have rated other services before and have completed a better profile for themselves. This may not go for the other rating sites, but I would be very careful and ask your patients to complete these things. It's a lot to ask, I know.

Emails to Follow-Up on Labs

I like to sit down with every patient and go over their labs in person. It is very confusing for them and the internet makes it even worse. "OMG, my RDW is a little off!" This, by the way, is why I don't think Big Tech will eliminate doctors or solve anything. There is too much room for interpretation of which labs are useful and which abnormalities are worth following up. After I meet with patients about their labs, I will then send a personalized email with recommendations. It is a macro I set up on my EMR that I tweak and individualize. Most of what I write has links for them to click on. In other words, I am trying to guide them to safer rabbit holes. Patients like this because they can never remember everything I said in the office and so they now can go over it on their own time and even email me with questions.

Get Deals for Your Patients

Consider getting your patients some bargains to other stores, professionals or services. You can even share discounts with these places. For example, maybe a massage/spa place nearby can offer a discount for your patients and you can offer a discount for theirs. This is another type of bartering, but it also gets the word out and gives your patients something tangible that they can actually use. How many other industries you can do this with is up to your imagination. It may be an accounting service, a restaurant, a local gym or CrossFit, and on and on. Patients also love the exclusive perks that only their doctor's office offers.

Give Your Patients Some Freebies

The concept of giving freebies never gets old. Another doc I know gives out free glucometers, which only cost him two cents each from McKesson. This may not be for everybody but the thought counts. We have free pens with our logo on it that we give away. We are also working on a bookmark that has some of my "health" recommendations on them. We also give free protein bars and water to anyone who gets labs done in our office. People love that, especially if they have been fasting.

Hook Into Their Technology

You can also find out what other products patients are using and hook into them. This can be an Apple watch or FitBit, where people can download their data right into their chart. Atlas.MD allows this to work seamlessly. It may be another service like Weight Watchers, where you can work with them to integrate their information to be shared with you. I hope to one day have a high tech or customized platform to get something of my service integrated into their daily lives. These things are a start.

Stay Current on Cool Stuff

Stay on top of new developments and tell patients about them. If you are doing something new in your office, then you want to tell patients about it. Brag about yourselves! For example, maybe it is a new liquid nitrogen gun for cryotherapy. Or, having a yoga instructor doing night classes in your office. Maybe it is new deep dive labs that are being offered, especially at a discounted price. Maybe it is new EKG machine or a procedure table. Maybe it is a course you took on hair restoration. It doesn't matter. You should always be thinking about new and cool things to add. Presently, we are looking into doing PRP injections. All this keeps you and your office fresh. It keeps you on your toes as well. Once you get it, make sure you announce it. Sharing these developments allows patients to share this with others and it also is another way to have a touch point with them so they don't forget you. Make it a press release for your patients via email or the newsletter. Or put it on FB. Cheesy? Who cares? Your patients need to know you are doing new things all the time. In fact, next time you go to a medical conference you should summarize what you learned and send it to patients in your newsletter or a mass email. Why? It explains why you needed to be out of the office for these things and shows that you are always learning. Patients love this.

Write a Weekly Newsletter

Right from the beginning I have been sending a weekly e-newsletter to all my patients via Constant Contact. It costs me $20 a month. My patients tell me they truly love it. In it there usually is one article about a research study that I discuss, a healthy food recipe, and then updates from our office. Why do I do this? Because it is a great reminder that I am still offering my patients something. It's just another touch point that I want them to fear losing if they quit the practice. I also want to own their "health news" and be the trusted curator of medical information out there in the sea of crap we are all seeing. All this gives them access to my unique perspective as a doctor. It gives them some insider knowledge that their friends and family are not getting. Other things that I occasionally put in there:

1. How we are still the best practice in town. We show examples but do it in a humble way
2. Highlight a business of a patient
3. Case studies of how we saved patients money
4. Special offers from other companies
5. Announcements of deals
6. Cross-selling and deals with other companies/professional
7. Reminders of the great reasons they are with us

Something else we are working on is a PDF of all the important items I put in the newsletters. We plan to give that away at the end of each year as a thank you gift. Remember, people love free things.

My engagement rate with these newsletters at or about 60%. This is a very good amount. Of course, I would like it to be higher but according to Constant Contact it is very impressive. I even got an award from them. Woo hoo. Actually, it was just a nice logo to put on my newsletter.

I do get great feedback from patients on my editorials and articles. It makes for good conversations about diet or HRT or whatever. I believe it is one of the most important and valued add-ons I offer to my patients.

Interestingly enough, I sometimes get lazy and forget to clear my Constant Contact newsletter list of people who do leave the practice. I recently found about 20 names and about 15 were still reading every newsletter. But alas they were deleted. Sorry folks, you have to pay to play.

Stay In Touch

Get in touch with "at risk" churners or those not using you. Some people are not using you enough, as I explained in an earlier chapter. I actually like it when patients come in for a yearly physical. And I don't care about what the experts say about these yearly exams. They base their opinions with cost in mind. For my patients, the labs are cheaper and the visits are included. In that vein, what we decided to do was use some of the analytics in my EMR (Atlas MD) to find out when each patient was seen last. The system creates a CSV file that I can play with on my Excel program. I easily sort out the people not seen the longest as well as others never seen! I couldn't believe it. People were paying me and never coming in. For each one of them, I worked methodically through it and sent them a personal email that I would like them to come in. Did it work for everyone? No. But it did for a lot and they just may stay longer due to that.

Throw a Party

Do an annual "Thank You" party in some manner. We do that with a Christmas party where one of our patients, who is a professional Santa actor, comes in for a couple of hours. This is very well attended, and people are so appreciative of it. It doesn't have to be a Christmas Party. It could be a New Year's Eve party or an anniversary party of when you opened. For that you may even get some press.

Start a Lecture Series

I mentioned this already, but I need to reiterate it here because it is very important. Do regular lectures for you patients on such topics as diet, workouts, cholesterol, etc. I have done this since I opened and even let the public come in. It's a marketing opportunity.

Connect People Together

Connect patients together with similar illnesses and do group patient meetings. It's funny but this is what they are doing in Great Britain because they just can't handle the volume in their National Health Service. But you're doing it as a way to truly educate and connect people.

Welcome Baskets for New Companies

When the staff of a Montessori school joined our practice, we did everything we could to give them great service. We really wanted to impress them. Business owners also talk to each other. Another thing we did was give them a big gift basket with:

- Almond snack packs
- Mini Larabars
- Stress balls with our logo
- Individual envelopes for each person with welcome letter containing pertinent contact info
- GoodRx cards
- Magnets with contact information on them
- Our gold cards
- Office brochures
- Office pens

We want to make them feel special and it cost us very little.

They Say It's Your Birthday

Each patient receives a personalized "Happy Birthday" email via my Atlas EMR. We were able to tweak the message, but the system takes care of the rest. Patients absolutely love it and they always thank us. It reminds them that we are thinking of them and anything that keeps us alive in their heads always helps to slow churn.

SECTION THREE:
SURVIVING

Chapter Fifteen:
Raising Your Rates and The Risk of Churn

A s I write this chapter, I have emailed my patients that I am raising their rates. I worried about this since I started my practice. After a full five years I decided to raise rates for new patients coming in. Then I gave my old patients eight months at their old rate and decided to bump everybody up to the new prices. My rates were $75 per month for a single, $125 per month for a couple and $150 per month for a family. We raised this to $80, $135, and $165 respectively. This was very tough for me to do as I always feared I would lose some patients. I asked other DPC docs what happened when they raised their rates, and they responded that very few left. I was still worried. What if a lot of mine left? Does that mean I am a bad doctor as compared to my peers? I held back sending the notice for months due to this fear. It's funny that no other business that I had dealt with feared sending me their rate increases. Every other expense I have kept going up in my five years in practice. Many went up multiple times. My rent goes up yearly. My accountant went up $25 a month on two different occasions. There was no reason I should feel bad about this other than I feared exposing myself and my insecurities. Maybe patients just won't feel like I'm worth it?

I researched every email that I could get on how to gently tell people I was going to raise their rates. I asked the other direct primary care doctors who I know for their letters and then searched the Internet for some templates. I looked at other subscription services to see what they wrote. After overthinking this, I decided on the following:

SUBJECT: Please read. Slight changes to Forest DPC

> After much careful consideration, we have made the decision to slightly raise our rates beginning on April 1, 2019. People who have joined since July 2018 have already been paying at our new rate, and we have been holding the prices for our other patients at the original rates since then. The prices will now be the same for all patients in our practice: $80 a month for a single, $135 a month for a couple and $165 a month for a family. (Please note this is the same rate that the new Boonsboro Direct Primary Care is also charging).

> Since starting Forest Direct Primary Care five years ago, we have made many improvements to our practice such as new lab testing options, cryotherapy and providing medical coverage through Dr. Anderson when I am away. Unfortunately, during this five-year period, each one of our expenses have increased, which forces us to make this slight increase in your rate.

> Our success would not have been possible without you and the investment in your health that you have made with us. We value our relationship with you and are

thankful for the trust you have placed in us. We are committed to giving you great service, and this slight increase will help us to do that.

If this price increase is a hardship for you, then please talk to me personally before deciding to leave and let's see if we can come up with a plan. I value your trust in me and would never want to lose that.

Sincerely,

Douglas Farrago MD

I had stomach pains in the morning as this went out. But maybe it wouldn't be so bad? Within minutes I received this:

Dr. F,

I appreciate the heads up. We will be one of the families leaving. I don't feel that we utilize enough of your services to justify the price we currently pay or an increase. Hopefully our leaving will open up a spot to a family that needs more of your time. What do I need to do in order to finalize this decision? I feel it would have been better to have sent this information out mid-month instead of the day your automatic draft comes out.

Thank you,

X

Ouch. I called this day Black Friday. But then I got this:

Dear Doctor F,

Your service is worth every penny and I am happy to pay the new rate.

Cheers,

Y

(Note: I thanked them for these kind words).

And then this from a family who I have been giving free care over the years:

Dr. Farrago,

Please start charging for my family. You have been more than generous, and it has been greatly appreciated. I don't know what we would have done without it.

Z

(Note: I still kept giving them free care)

And then this:

Thanks for letting us know! Still.. 100% WORTH IT!!

And this:

Good morning,

Thank you for providing such good care for our family. We appreciate you and your staff. We really enjoy being patients of FDPC.

We certainly understand your rate increase being necessary for your practice. As a self-employed business owner, I can appreciate where you're coming from with cost of business increasing.

Since XXXX lost his job in the beginning of January, we've been re-evaluating all of our expenses during this unexpected financially difficult season. We are wondering if it would be possible to maintain our current rate of $150 for the next 3 months and then re-evaluate from there? We're hoping in the next 3 months our financial situation will improve as he continues to pursue new job opportunities.

Let me know if that might be an option for FDPC.

Thanks,

We obviously obliged this family.

I spoke to some of my DPC peers and buddies about this worry of mine. Here are some of their responses:

- We went up by $10/mo for individuals, and proportionately for couples and families (about 20%). We did this for everyone at once, established and new, about 9 months ago. (My wife/office manager grandfathered most of the over 65 yo crowd whether they needed the discount or not.) I think we had a total of 2 or 3 leave out of over 600. I will tell you that those who left were always complaining about our fees all the time anyway. They did not appreciate us from the start. We were happy to see them go. That made room for new patients who value what we do. I am sure you will have the same experience

- I am getting ready to do the same thing. That is a very reasonable increase, especially after so long. Even with the people leaving, you'll have less work and more money, or same work and more money if you add people to replace them. I just went to get my hair cut, and the person who cuts my hair, who is in her early 20s, let me know that she has gotten a "promotion" and that it will now cost $50 for me to get my hair cut by her, which takes her maybe 20 mins. That is my average price per MONTH of medical care. I am willing to pay her that because she does a good job and I like her, and I hope that most of your patients and my patients will be willing to pay an increase too.

- We raised our rates by $5-10 for most (kids and >60 stayed the same) at our 3-year anniversary. Had a handful leave, but most didn't bat an eye. Those who left were just needing an excuse and we were happy to oblige.

- Never take it personally. People view us/our practices solely as a financial decision. No matter how great we are or what loyalty they profess, it comes down to $$. The nice thing is for every person who leaves over a price increase, there are 2 others waiting to jump in because they hate the hamster wheel. On we go. Another day in DPC. Still WAY better than the alternative.

By 10 AM a few more left. I had done a few cosmetic skin tag/ mole removals on one of these patients only a week earlier. It easily would have cost her $500 out of pocket elsewhere. She was happy as a clam when she left that day but for $5 more per month, she gave us a two-line email, "Hey can you please discontinue my membership? Thank you!!". And poof, she was gone. Be well.

The other one that left on this day did give a nice thank you and explained that this was a strain for her anyway. I got the sense she truly valued our services and maybe that is all I really wanted. I am human. Doctors are human. It still sucks when you put your heart and soul into your practice and into your patient relationships and they just vanish for $5 a month.

Due to the way my payment model is set up I had to go through all my patients by hand and change them to their new rates. I created some shortcuts to make it easier by looking at the head of each family instead of each individual member, but I still had to go through every single member. It was a pain in the butt, but I was able to find patients I haven't seen in a while and personally emailed them to schedule a physical and got some responses! Even better, I found one patient who wasn't billed for four months and another for 20 months! Both paid up. I made $1800 because of this. Nothing like finding that twenty-dollar bill in the pocket of that old jacket you put on.

Overall, we lost about 10 patients at most. Some waited a month, but I am sure it was due to the increase. More importantly, it is over now, and I am at peace with it.

Chapter Sixteen:
The Four Agreements of DPC

Sometimes there is nothing you can do to totally stop the churn. Yes, you should work hard, do your best each day and keep learning how to be a better doctor business owner. But, after that, you need to let go. Let me talk about *The Four Agreements: A Practical Guide to Personal Freedom (A Toltec Wisdom Book)* by Don Miguel Ruiz at this time because it works well in life and maybe even better for direct primary care. Here they are:

1. Be impeccable with your word
2. Don't take anything personally
3. Don't make assumptions
4. Always do your best

The first agreement explains why keeping your word to your patients and to yourself is critical. It's about keeping your promises, and no specialty in healthcare works better for all this than doing direct primary care. I think we are so less conflicted than we used to be in the FFS model. So, there is not much to say about this one.

Let me skip to the fourth agreement. Always do your best. Without the bureaucratic drag of the system and administrators holding us back, I am sure you are on top of this one as well. I know so many DPC docs now and they are happy, altruistic human beings. These are good people who just needed the right environment so they could do their best and feel appreciated for doing it. There are times, however, that even in DPC you will feel overwhelmed. Even the subject of this book, churn, will break you at times. All you can do is your best. At least you are reading this and working on things. Other doctors in the system are robotic and trying to just get through their days without killing themselves. Literally. You need to get to the point that even if six families leave your practice in a week, you still know you will be ok. It is what it is. Learn from it and continue to do your best.

Now the hard part. The middle two agreements are critical for surviving as a DPC doc. Don't assume anything and don't take anything personal. Yes, at times it will be difficult. You need to get some thick skin here and let things go. It doesn't mean you are emotionless. It just means you are not going to waste your emotions and drain your energy because some patients leave your practice. You will learn but you will not burn. Let me tell you how.

Is That So?

In Eckhart Tolle's book *A New Earth: Awakening To Your Life's Purpose*, he tells a story about a Zen master to illustrate an important lesson. You can read that version online, or in his book, but I tweaked it and twisted it around to make it applicable for a DPC practice. Here goes:

A direct primary care doctor lived in a small town in Virginia. He was held in high regard and many people came to him for their care. Then it happened that a patient quit his practice because he felt he could no longer afford or needed it. He told the doctor this one day in the office.

The DPC doctor replied, "Is that so?"

The patient stated "yes" even though he spends more on his cable bill, cell phone carrier, a food delivery service, a gym membership that he never uses and on and on.

The doctor smiled and explained to him that it is his choice what he values and told him to "Be Well".

The DPC doctor never thought of that patient again. He remained unfazed and went about being a great doctor to his other patients. Sometime later, when the DPC doctor saw the same patient at the health food store, the patient asked how his practice was. The DPC doctor replied, "Great! I love treating and helping people who value my service".

The patient was taken a little off guard and replied, "Is that so?" The doctor nodded his head yes.

A year later that same patient saw the doctor and asked if he could rejoin the practice. "Is that so?" replied the DPC doctor.

"Yes, I really can't get in to see my other doctor and he doesn't seem to care anyway."

The DPC doctor replied, "Is that so?"

The patient said yes and asked when he could get in.

"Well, I have a waiting list now so just give your name to my receptionist and we will call when there is an opening".

The patient replied, "Is that so?" The doctor said yes and told him to call his office to get on that list.

And they never saw each other again.

Here is Eckhart Tolle's commentary on the original Hakuin's Zen Story that I tweaked to a DPC parable:

> "The story of the Zen Master whose only response was always "Is that so?" shows the good that comes through inner nonresistance to events, that is to say, being at one with what happens.....Nonresistance, non-judgement, and non-attachment are the three aspects of true freedom and enlightened living."

Does this make sense? You may have to think about this for a bit. The DPC doctor never emotionally got caught up in why the patient left. He never assumed anything or took anything personal. It's the patient's loss, as he is the one who left, and the DPC doctor just continued to do his best. The patient had his own story and his own excuses, and in the end, will have to pay for it.

So, when patients give you some lame excuse why they can't join, or why they need to leave, remember that it is their journey. Don't get caught up in it. Don't assume anything or take it personally. Just say "Is that so?" and then give them a nice "Be Well".

Be Well

I am pretty famous, or infamous, in the direct primary care world over my "Be Well" response. Sounds stupid but it's not. It's cathartic. What does it really mean? Well, when I decided to do DPC here in Virginia there was a local group trying to hire me. I was offered a job by them a few years earlier but couldn't pull the trigger. I wasn't interested in working in the system anymore, but a year later I did some work for them as an independent contractor. When that job ended, and they had no other job to offer me, I sent a nice long and warm letter to the head guy. I thanked him and told him about how I wanted to be the doctor I always dreamed of being. I told him I was going to jump in head first and be the first DPC doctor in the area. It wasn't personal. It was the system that was broken. It was a long heart felt email and a very appreciative one. His only response to me, pouring my guts out, was two words: "Be Well".

It threw me for a loop. It made me think for days. Two words? And then I realized what he was saying with "Be Well" was...."Go f%ck yourself". I got it. He said it without saying it. And I am sure he felt satisfaction inside. I really have no ill will towards him for that. It was actually brilliant. Where am I going with this? Well, I took it as a lesson. Those patients who leave to save a few dollars for worse care in the FFS model get a "Be Well" from me. Or those patients, who leave after overusing and abusing me with tons of appointments, get a "Be Well" from me. Or those patients who complain about something ridiculous, when I know it really is about money, and then leave get the same "Be Well" from me. No long responses to their email. Do I fight them point by point? No. Do ask them why they are leaving? No. My staff may but not me. All I do is answer with two words: "Be Well". And only I know, in my heart, what that means. And it feels so good inside and makes the hurt a little bit less. Now that I told you my secret, try it. Try it with your next patient who leaves, after you did so much for them, and see if this doesn't help soothe you.

By the way, this does NOT mean that when you say "Be Well" it is always a bad thing. That is up to you. Sometimes YOU REALLY MEAN it in a nice and genuine way. It's your choice and only you know.

This little trick has helped so many people in the DPC world that I even had t-shirts made. Yup, I went out and paid someone to draw my Physician "Be Well" Series. You can see them on dpcbook.com. Feel free to purchase one and see if you can tell whether the raised finger is the middle one or not.

Chapter Seventeen:
You Are Not an Imposter

Okay, we are starting to get close to the end, so I need to pump you up. How do I know? Because I need pumping up.....a lot. One thing you have to remember is that DPC is a better job than any other primary care option out there. It's not even close. The problem is that being a doctor is still hard at times and DPC just has its own new and distinct issues. For one, DPC is a lonely sport. Most of us are solo docs. As awesome as it is to be in full control, and an owner of your own business, there is still an isolation issue. Not having other docs as your peers to talk with in person can be tough. You should not complain or commiserate to your MA, nurse or assistant. It just looks bad. So, most of us hold it in and unfortunately it wears us down.

Another issue specific to DPC is feeling that you are not adequate enough at times. All of us have good intentions yet many of us also know that we are not always right. That sliver of doubt can grow in DPC to the point where you start questioning yourself. You start thinking, "Why are these people even listening to me?" or "Do I know what I'm doing?". I've been through this. It gets worse when you have some complaints come your way or people start leaving the practice. I am here to tell you that this is normal. It's an occupational risk in the DPC profession. It's called "Imposter Syndrome". Here is what Wikipedia says about it:

> Imposter syndrome (also known as imposter phenomenon, imposterism, fraud syndrome or the impostor experience) is a psychological pattern in which an individual doubts their accomplishments and has a persistent internalized fear of being exposed as a "fraud". Despite external evidence of their competence, those experiencing this phenomenon remain convinced that they are frauds, and do not deserve all they have achieved. Individuals with imposterism incorrectly attribute their success to luck, or as a result of deceiving others into thinking they are more intelligent than they perceive themselves to be. While early research focused on the prevalence among high-achieving women, impostor syndrome has been recognized to affect both men and women equally.

This is really an issue of confidence. I am always amazed when I see those with the most education and most experience still doubt themselves. Part of this is a good thing so that we keep learning. Mostly, it can be a downer and can make you lose confidence in yourself. Once that happens, patients will feel it and may start to leave.

Let's compare that to those less educated and less trained who are entering the medical field, even DPC, feeling like they are fully prepared. I see the Dunning-Kruger effect over and over again. What's that? In 1999 psychologist David Dunning, and his graduate student Justin Kruger, published a paper about a phenomenon where:

> The most competent individuals tend to underestimate their relative ability a little, but for most people (the bottom 75%) they increasingly overestimate their ability,

and everyone thinks they are above average. There are several possible causes of the effect. One is simple ego – no one wants to think of themselves as below average, so they inflate their self-assessment. People also have an easier time recognizing ignorance in others than in themselves, and this will create the illusion that they are above average, even when they are in the single digits of percentile.

Dunning said that, "Incompetent people do not recognize—scratch that, cannot recognize—just how incompetent they are. What's curious is that, in many cases, incompetence does not leave people disoriented, perplexed, or cautious. Instead, the incompetent are often blessed with an inappropriate confidence, buoyed by something that feels to them like knowledge."
Neurologica Blog 11/6/14

To summarize, you are good enough. You are more than good enough. As a trained and board-certified primary care doctor you are what DPC patients need. You are not an imposter. This is not to say there aren't imposters out there, however. There are many who pretend to be as good as a doctor/physician and even try to use the "doctor" title. Unfortunately, due to their lack of training, as compared to ours, they do not know what they do not know and are somehow "buoyed by something that feels like knowledge" but it isn't. This means that they are not being open and honest with patients and we need to have a public discussion about the difference between real doctors versus imposters. Why? Because this group (NPs mostly are trying to do DPC on their own) has chosen not to collaborate with us, but has chosen to compete with us and to do so for a cheaper price. They do this while claiming they are equal to doctors based on industry-supported, biased research studies, that were created with the intent on confirming their bias. Please read the following:

As an older 2nd career med student/former Psych NP, I don't agree with the push for FPA and I absolutely disagree with their contention that NPs are equal to MDs. Having been an NP and graduating as an MD in a few weeks, this is so untrue. The education of NP barley scratches the surface of MD education. The original intent of NP was not to be equal nor replace MDs, but it was to augment MD tasks assigned on physician led teams. It has now morphed into an ugly juggernaut. Now there is even role hijacking with NPs claiming to practice medicine and that is their new role now despite MDs already doing this. I often ask when did it become ok for one discipline to take the role of another discipline and claim it to be their own despite the original discipline already doing these roles? It's not right and MDs need to push back. In psychiatry, my NP education pales in comparison to my MD education, and I haven't even done residency yet. Diploma mills with watered down, poor quality programs and the rush of inexperienced RNs to apply to these programs are part to blame.

I agree with him. We need to fight this. This does not mean I am anti-NP or anti-PA. I have many who I am friends with and respect tremendously. I am just against the extremist ones who perpetuate the lie that training and education do not matter. It does, and we should, as physicians, be offended by their attacks.

So where does this leave us. Well, most of you are out there on your own and will definitely doubt yourself now and then. Please don't. Listen to Rocky. Here is his motivational speech to his son from the movie Rocky Balboa (2006):

"Let me tell you something you already know. The world ain't all sunshine and rainbows. It's a very mean and nasty place and I don't care how tough you are it will beat you to your knees and keep you there permanently if you let it. You, me, or nobody is gonna hit as hard as life. But it ain't about how hard ya hit. It's about how hard you can get hit and keep moving forward. How much you can take and keep moving forward. That's how winning is done! Now if you know what you're worth then go out and get what you're worth. But ya gotta be willing to take the hits, and not pointing fingers saying you ain't where you wanna be because of him, or her, or anybody! Cowards do that and that ain't you! You're better than that! I'm always gonna love you no matter what. No matter what happens. You're my son and you're my blood. You're the best thing in my life. But until you start believing in yourself, ya ain't gonna have a life. "

Start believing in yourself or ya ain't gonna have a life.

Chapter Eighteen: Conclusion

I hope this book has been helpful for you. If you save even one patient from leaving, then it is worth almost 50 times what you paid for it. My hope is that you do not ignore this issue. You don't want to sail across the Atlantic with a leaky boat. The first step is the awareness that churn can be an issue. But, hey, maybe you are lucky, and it is not an issue for you. Great. But times change. The landscape of medicine, and DPC, is always changing and if you are not on top of this then it will end up biting you in the ass.

I will end this with a few "coincidental" patient encounters. The first was a recent meet-and-greet of a woman who really was on point with her questions. She knew exactly what she wanted to ask and realized that I was also interviewing her. Then she asked, "What is your churn rate?" Wow. Smart woman. She figured out that a high churn rate may be a problem with my practice or DPC in general. I was honest with her and told her my numbers. I told her that the newness of DPC adds to the churn but there are a ton of other factors. We also don't have great benchmarks. It was a nice conversation and she eventually joined the practice. What will you say when a prospective patient asks you your churn rate?

Another situation also made me ponder my career. I was recently onboarding a business and their ten employees. I was doing some backend work to get their names on my newsletter. As I was doing this I was talking to my wife and feeling really proud of myself and the practice. At that very moment an email came in with a patient cancelling their services. And it wasn't a nice one. The lesson: never get too cocky or complacent. This job won't let you.

Lastly, as I finish this book, I want to tell you about a couple of patients who just left. They had been with me for nine months. I had seen them both a combined 8 or 9 times. Their labs were off, the husband was on a ton of meds, and I was able to motivate them to both lose weight. We kept them accountable with follow ups, their labs normalized and they came off their meds. They seemed so happy. They were treated like gold every time they came in. Heck, they came to our Christmas party and brought their grandkids. And then they emailed to say they were going back to their previous doctor due to "not having a comfort level" with me. WTF? Really? Now I looked over their charts. I mentally went over their visits. I know the wife had a scowl on her face at times. She seemed to be judging me, but the husband was so happy. And their outcomes were great. Before I let my ego get involved, I just decided to move on. I did not email them to ask why. I archived their charts and asked other patients from the waiting list to join. Be well. Sometimes there is no rhyme or reason to the churn.

So, let me end with this. I earlier mentioned Steve Martin's line when trying to market yourself. "Be so good they can't ignore you". Let me tweak this for slowing the DPC churn. I would say also "Be so good they can't forget you and then remind them over and over again."

Post script:

Our office won the Bedford County Chamber of Commerce Small Business of the Year Award. We were all there to receive this high honor. There were over 200 business owners at this formal event, and we were so honored when one of my patients and board members presented it to us. That night was a high for all of us and the next morning we had a meeting to discuss how to dispense the news to our patients as well as market it to new potential members. A few hours later a patient called to cancel their membership. The reasons? Well, they love my assistant because she literally spent hours and hours doing referrals for them. So, what was it? The money, they said, was becoming an issue. But...... the husband also had to throw in that I chastised the wife on her last visit. That visit was almost a year ago. At that time, she walked in to the office while other patients were there, wanting to be seen for a non-urgent issue. I did see her but asked her nicely to please call ahead of time in the future because it's not fair to the patients with scheduled appointments. She obviously was angry at that. The husband also said that he did not appreciate my emails because they did not have the niceties they should have. So, which reason was it? Well, it's always the money. The rest was just rationalization so they could feel good about their decision. Don't get me wrong, I can be better. We all can. Mostly this showed me not to get too high, even after winning an award, because sooner or later someone is going to knock you in the crotch.

I never said this stuff was easy. Because it never is.

Be well.

Appendix A:
Stages of Churn Grief

Okay, as I am writing this a husband and wife just emailed me. The subject line was "Cancelling Services". My first thought was "Son-of-a-bitch". The following are the stages you will probably go through when a patient leaves your practice. Remember, this is new and didn't probably happen to you in the FFS model. DPC is different and keeping in line with Elisabeth Kübler-Ross, here you go:

1. Denial – No way. They like it here. Must be a mistake. They seemed so appreciative. Is that right? I'm confused.

2. Anger – That's bullshit. I worked so hard for that patient/family. Did they just use me? I never liked them, anyway. She always had an attitude. He was disrespectful at times.

3. Bargaining – I wonder what I can do to make them stay? Maybe I should email them and ask what I could have done differently.

4. Depression – This is such a bummer. I worked so hard to onboard them and now they are gone. Maybe I suck as a doctor.

5. Acceptance – Screw it, I'm a good doctor. It's on them if they leave. I cannot do better or care more. Some people just don't fit in this style of practice. Be well.

If you are new you may think this strange or funny. You can laugh all you want. Ignore it or put this away, but you will need to look at it someday. Remember me, which will be the future you, when someone who you never thought would leave quits out of the blue. When that happens remember that there is a good chance you will go through these stages just like we all do. And it's going to be okay.

Appendix B:
The DPC Family

One of the toughest things I had to deal with is unfair competition. It threw me for a loop and I didn't know why. It seems a doctor, at the time of this writing, is trying steal my patients by converting his FFS practice into a DPC hybrid practice. I have no problem with anyone going into DPC. I have said that over and over again in my first book. I hope this phenomenon changes how medicine is practiced. A rising tide floats all boats. We are all in this together.

But what if there is a wrench in this "family" mentality? The doctor, who has chosen to compete with me, is only about a quarter of a mile away. That's kind of close but he bought the facility, and to be fair, that FFS building was there before me. Here's where it gets tricky. He never talked to me. He did talk to the DPC doc across town, who I spent countless hours helping to open up his practice. I found that weird. Then I saw the billboards advertising his practice. These billboards, co-incidentally enough, were right in front of the office park where I am located. Wow, I thought, that's a little aggressive. Then I saw his prices. My jaw dropped. His monthly rate was 25% lower than mine for one person. He cut his family rate to the point that it would be half of what I charge. This person was trying to steal my patients.

I had to speak with a few of my DPC friends to vent. Their response was, "His model is unsustainable financially". They are right and they didn't even know how big his building or staff is. I do and it is huge. The only way for him to make a decent living, with these rates, would be to double the number of patients he has. This all goes against the DPC model. He is doing this by trying to convert as many of his own FFS patients as well as stealing whomever he can from me.

I understand, all is fair in love and war. And I guess the same goes for business and direct primary care. You will have competition someday, too. It's coming. When I wrote my first book, I never thought it would be this fast and I never thought of the types of competition ahead. There are tons of "entrepreneurs" trying to get into the game. There are VC backed DPC franchises coming. There are hospitals dipping their toes in the game. I suspect the health insurers are coming next. So, what do we do? Hell, what do I do?

Before I get to my answer, I want to discuss the biggest problem with the doctor who chose to go after my patients and hurt me in order for him to succeed. What he did, in my mind, is disrupt the family atmosphere around DPC. He chose never to talk to me. This was obviously on purpose. I know I am but a speck in this big planet, but I am pretty well known in the DPC world, as small as it is. I started DPC in my community. This doctor also chose to be very aggressive in his pricing, to the point where it changes how many patients he will need to have in the practice in order to make a living. But the biggest issue I have is that instead of being a colleague he was a coward. Instead of trying to be a friend he has chosen to go to war and hurt me. This, probably more than anything else, just makes me sad.

As you try and tweak your practice to make it better, please understand that DPC is a brotherhood and sisterhood. We are all in this together. Be nice. Be friendly. Play fair. There are so many others out there who are trying to stop the incredible progress that we made, we don't need to cannibalize each other. No one is asking that you collude to keep all the prices the same as the next DPC doctor. I am surely not saying that. But going to half the rate for families, as the jerk did down the block, was beyond reasonable.

All I can do now is be the best DPC doctor I can be for my patients. Even though I wrote this and two other DPC books, it doesn't matter. I still need to read it over and over again. I need to constantly evaluate what I can do better. I need to constantly see what "broken windows" I have. I need to constantly look for opportunities to give better value to my patients.

The weirdest irony is that no one needs this book on "churn" more than I do right now because of the unfair competition that has come my way. By the time you read this I could be out of business. But as Melisandre asked Ayra at the Battle of Winterfell, in the Game of Thrones, "What do we say to the God of Death?".

Ayra response was, "Not today".

The same goes for me.

Not today.

Appendix C:
Welcome to the Practice Email

Dear (name):

I just wanted to welcome you to the practice. Forest Direct Primary Care is the first of its kind in central Virginia. We pride ourselves in providing great service, transparent pricing and excellent medical care. Some things you should know about the practice:

1. We can get you in pretty shortly for any acute problem that you may have. Just call us at (434) 616-2455. We do complete annual physicals on everyone. They are scheduled 4 to 6 weeks out because these require an initial hour-long appointment with a half hour follow-up. Please call Christine at the number above to set this up. Christine Creasey is Dr. Farrago's assistant in the office and her responsibilities include phlebotomy, scheduling, assisting with procedures, making referrals, answering calls and taking vital signs. She has been with us since the opening of the office.

2. Debbie Farrago, Dr. Farrago's wife, is the office manager and helps with many of the things behind the scenes including all business affairs.

3. Dr. Farrago is your primary care doctor who answers all emails directed to forestdpc@gmail.com. He will be the doctor seeing you unless it is one of the few days he takes off for a conference or a vacation. He still answers his email and questions from Christine.

4. Dr. Anderson at Boonsboro Direct Primary Care covers for Dr. Farrago when he is out and Dr. Farrago does the same for him. If you need to be seen when Dr. Farrago is out, Christine will call Dr. Anderson's office to get that appointment for you. This visit is still FREE of charge.

5. You do not need to arrive at your appointment early. Just come at the scheduled time.

6. We would like for you to come in for a physical once a year, and it would help if you keep a reminder of when you are due each year. Just call the office at your convenience to schedule this.

7. We try to have one party every year to recognize how much we appreciate our patients. We sure hope you come.

8. Labs are not included in your monthly fee. That being said, we pass the discounted prices we get from the lab companies on to you. Dr. Farrago does in depth labs and he usually orders these at the time of your physical.

9. We believe all patients are equal. Everyone deserves their own 30-60 minutes that they have scheduled with Dr. Farrago. Please don't stop in for a quick visit unannounced. It is not that we don't like you or don't want to see you but, it is unfair to the other person in the office seeing Dr. Farrago. We pretty much guarantee to get you in the day you need to be seen so please just call ahead to schedule a time.

10. We do like to follow up closely for any chronic medical problems so please show up for your appointments. You will get email or text reminders for you scheduled appointments.

11. Dr. Farrago will talk to you a lot about lifestyle changes such as exercise and diet and he tries to keep you accountable. Do not take this personally. This is what doctors are supposed to do.

12. Please open and read the weekly newsletter every Wednesday. In the newsletter is important information about the office, great recipes and analyses by Dr. Farrago of current medical topics.

13. Dr. Farrago will be lecturing every few months. These topics include diet, exercise, etc. We sure hope you come.

14. Twice a year, the Centra Mammography Van comes right to our office as a benefit to our patients.

15. After hours or on weekends you can call Dr. Farrago (xxx-xxxx) if you have a critical issue. If you have an issue that is not critical, you may email him anytime at forestdpc@ gmail.com with your question. If you have a life-threatening situation, please call 911.

16. We are happy you have joined our practice, and we hope to have a long-lasting relationship with you! If, for some reason you need to leave our office, please note that per our contract we require a 30-day notice.

Douglas Farrago and the Staff at Forest Direct Primary Care

Appendix D:
Sample Newsletter

Your Weekly Office News & Health Updates

Sugar is Sugar

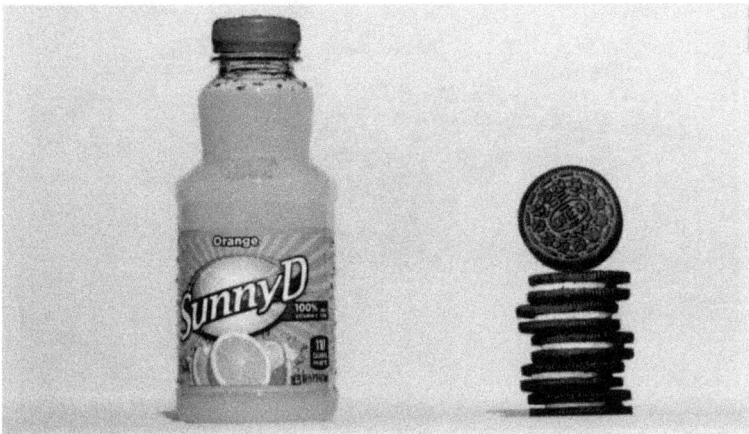

Here is an interesting article in CNN. It turns out that fruit juice is basically sugar. I think we all knew that but we sometimes convince ourselves that it is really healthy for us. But is it? Or was it the producers of fruit juice who figured out a perfect marketing plan. Well, here is some information:

- Specifically, drinking an excessive amount of fruit juice could lead to an increased risk of premature death ranging from 9% to 42%, according to the study, published Friday in the journal JAMA Network Open.

- Overall, the sugars found in orange juice, although naturally occurring, are pretty similar to the sugars added to soda and other sweetened beverages, the study suggests.

The study also reinforces the evidence behind carbs being a major culprit in heart disease.

My take: Carbs are an issue. They are addictive and they cause health problems. You just need to keep an eye on them and limit them, even in fruit or fruit juices. Oh, and you need to click on the link above and see the pictures comparing different drinks to sugary foods. It is at the bottom.

PROTEIN FIBER CRACKERS

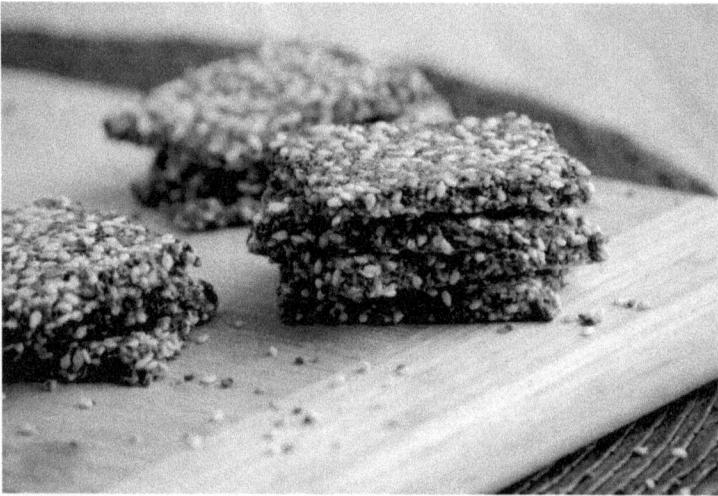

Ingredients:

1/2 cup sesame seeds

1/2 cup chia seeds

1/4 cup flaxseed meal

1/4 cup almond meal

1/2 tsp salt

1/3 cup water

2 tbsp extra virgin olive oil

Instructions:

1. Preheat the oven to 325 degrees F. In a large bowl, mix together the sesame seeds, chia seeds, flaxseed meal, almond meal, and salt. Mix in the water and olive oil until combined.

2. Transfer the dough to a sheet of parchment paper. Cover with a second sheet of paper and roll out the dough to 1/4-inch thick. Peel back the top layer of paper and cut the dough into squares.

3. Place the parchment paper with the squares onto a baking sheet. Bake for 30 minutes, and then use a spatula to carefully flip over. Bake for an additional 25-30 minutes until lightly browned. Let cool for 30 minutes before serving.

Servings: 9-12 crackers

LINK

OFFICE UPDATE

Medicare Patients: Even though we do not file any claims with Medicare or any other insurance, we still like to have your card on file for referrals. The government is issuing new Medicare cards with a new identification number. They will no longer contain your social security which makes your identity more secure. Once you receive your new card in the mail, please make sure you bring it with you to your next appointment so that we can update our records. We thank you for your assistance with this.

Quick Notes:

If you are traveling and need vaccines, here is some info:

https://www.cdc.gov/features/vaccines-travel/index.html

Here is a good article on Measles:

https://www.newsadvance.com/news/trending/how-does-measles-spread-do-i-need-another-mmr-vaccine/article_4f2b3bf3-692a-53a4-906a-225b4f7d237c.html

As far as contacting me:

- CALL 911 for emergencies
- At night, call my cell if this an emergency but not enough to call 911
- Use texting for urgent matters not basic questions
- Use email if things can wait as they may not be answered for 24 hours.
- I do not look at email or texts after 9 PM so you must call then if it is critical

Important Numbers:

The office number is XXX-xxxx

My personal cell is xxx-xxxx

Christine's email is _____

My email is _____

Thanks for reading our newsletter and email me with any questions.

Douglas Farrago MD

Appendix E:
Sample Email Follow-Up After Discussing Labs

*Obviously, this reflects my personal health biases. Your opinions may differ. That's totally fine. Copy whatever you want. By the time you read this I may have changed my mind about certain things and switched references, but you get the point.

Dear (name):

It was great speaking with you today. Your labs show that you are at the fork in the road in life. It's up to you which direction you go. So, here are my thoughts:

1. Your LDL-P and small LDL are up and your HDL-P is low. Here is a site for reference: https://www.labcorp.com/tests/related-documents/L15035

2. Your vitamin D is low. I am not sure if supplementation is the right way to go. Read this:

3. https://www.sciencealert.com/vitamin-d-tablets-may-be-worse-for-you-then-nothing-at-all

4. Your testosterone is not optimal which all means an inflammatory lifestyle (diet, exercise, poor sleep).

5. Most diets are fine as long as carbs are controlled. As a good guideline, I recommend you watch the Paleo Diet video here:

   https://www.youtube.com/watch?list=UUfvZUb-mQZ6OQjaGyR8M36SA&v=BhZqIaTprjk

   but also get The Paleo Solution:

   http://www.amazon.com/Paleo-Solution-Original-Human-Diet/dp/0982565844/ref=sr_1_1?ie=UTF8&qid=1421951068&sr=8-1&keywords=the+paleo+solution

*Ignore his supplement recommendations, however, as they are outdated and wrong.

6. Also, there is great information on what is called Time Restricted Eating. See these videos of Rhonda Patrick. Be warned that Joe Rogan can swear a bit:

   https://www.youtube.com/watch?v=0UqxC2RDF64

   https://www.youtube.com/watch?v=zz4YVJ4aRfg

7. Everyone should understand a little about circadian rhythms and light. Read this:

   http://www.health.harvard.edu/staying-healthy/blue-light-has-a-dark-side

8. You may need to cut the blue light out with blue blockers and Just Get Flux. Here are links:

   http://www.amazon.com/Uvex-S1933X-Eyewear-SCT-Orange-Anti-Fog/dp/B000USRG90/ref=sr_1_3?ie=UTF8&qid=1421765232&sr=8-3&keywords=blue+blockers

   and

   https://justgetflux.com

9. Enjoy nature, go barefoot and touch the ground daily (more on that another day)

10. Get some sun early in the morning each day. This will actually help your sleep later.

11. Follow your carbs by using Myfitnesspal app and keep them under 100 grams a day and don't eat after 6 PM!

12. Take your body weight and divide it in half and drink that many ounces of non-fluoridated water a day (like spring water).

13. Everyone should be exercising 4-5 times a week. This NEEDS to include both cardio (walking, elliptical, running, etc.) and resistance training (lifting weights). These two

things make people LIVE LONGER!

14. Your homocysteine is up a little. Here is a site for reference:

    http://www.drweil.com/drw/u/ART03423/Elevated-Homocysteine.html

15. Your hemoglobin A1C is up and this is also related to carbohydrate intake so see the diet and carb gram recommendations above.

    https://labtestsonline.org/understanding/analytes/a1c/tab/test/

16. Your Lp (a) was high. Lipoprotein(a), is a particle in your blood which carries cholesterol, fats and proteins. The amount your body makes is inherited from one or both parents and is determined by the genes passed on from your parent(s) when you are born. It does not change very much during your lifetime except if you are a woman, levels increase as the natural estrogen level declines with menopause. Diet and exercise seem to have little to no impact on the lipoprotein(a) level. It does increase your risk of heart disease. Read more here:

    https://www.nytimes.com/2018/01/09/well/heart-risk-doctors-lipoprotein.html

    http://www.lipoproteinafoundation.org/?page=UnderstandLpa

    The drugs for this are new and you would need to ask your insurance about them:

    https://www.drugs.com/slideshow/pcsk9-inhibitors-a-new-option-in-cholesterol-treatment-1166

17. Sleep

    a. Improving Your Sleep:

       https://www.alexfergus.com/blog/how-to-improve-your-sleep-with-morning-sunlight

b. Another article

http://www.huffingtonpost.com/dr-michael-tolen-tino/the-blue-light-threat-to-_b_9853562.html

c. Podcast: These THREE episodes on sleep were amazing. The first one is here:

https://peterattiamd.com/matthewwalker1/

THERE ARE THREE EPISODES. LISTEN TO THEM ALL. BUY THE BOOK.

18. Your Omega 6 to Omega 3 ratio is off. It should be in the 4 to 1 range. For most people that is due to too many Omega 6s and too little Omega 3s. This increases the chance of obesity. Read this:

http://www.endocrinologyadvisor.com/obesity/omega-6-to-omega-3-fatty-acid-ratio-plays-role-in-obesity/article/568452/

Also, here is a link to understand which foods have which:

http://fanaticcook.blogspot.com/2009/04/omega-6-and-omega-3-in-foods.html

DHA is your most important Omega-3 and that comes in seafood. The smaller the fish the better (ex. sardines). They say you need about 5 seafood meals a week, but it can be just some sardines.

The highest amount of DHA is in SMASH:

Sardines

Mackerel

Anchovies

Salmon

Herring

plus mollusk and shellfish

If you CANNOT eat seafood, then try:

https://www.amazon.com/Viva-Naturals-Krill-Oil-Antarctic/dp/B004TBCT4G/ref=sr_1_4_s_it?s=hpc&ie=UTF8&qid=1522161752&sr=1-4&keywords=krill+oil

or if you are vegetarian

https://www.amazon.com/Nordic-Naturals-Health-Optimal-Wellness/dp/B009KTUGSS/ref=sr_1_1_a_it?ie=UTF8&qid=1490900901&sr=8-1&keywords=algae+omega+nordic+naturals

Keep reading my health updates as they come out as well

You will have questions so just email them to me.

Thanks,

Dr. Farrago

Appendix F:
The Direct Primary Care Alliance

I have to ask you a favor. Please consider joining the Direct Primary Care Alliance. This organization was started by the best people, I believe, in the DPC world. The Direct Primary Care Alliance (DPCA) is a grassroots organization providing vision, leadership, and guidance to the DPC community through physician-led education, mentorship, advocacy, and organizational intelligence. No doctor is being paid for the hours and hours of work he or she has put in. It is already becoming the voice for questions about direct primary care and the go-to for the media. We don't want other organizations speaking for us. The yearly fee is nominal and the benefits are many including those listed above as well as tremendous discounts for purchases you make regularly for you office. For more information, go to www.dpcalliance.org.

About the Author

Douglas Farrago, MD received his Bachelor of Science from the University of Virginia in 1987, his Masters of Education degree in the area of Exercise Science from the University of Houston in 1990, and his Medical Degree from the University of Texas at Houston in 1994. His residency training occurred way up north at the Eastern Maine Medical Center in Bangor, Maine. In his final year, he was elected Chief Resident by his peers. Dr. Farrago has practiced family medicine for twenty-three years, first in Auburn, Maine and now in Forest, Virginia. He founded Forest Direct Primary Care in 2014, which quickly filled in 18 months. Dr. Farrago invented the Knee Saver, a padding that relieves knee stress in baseball catchers, while he was in medical school. The original Knee Saver is currently in the Baseball Hall of Fame. He is also the inventor of the Cryohelmet worn by people for migraines, heat recovery and head injuries. Dr. Farrago created the Placebo Journal in 2001 and ran it until 2011. His first book, the Placebo Chronicles, was published by Broadway Books. Dr. Farrago still blogs every day on his website Authentic-medicine.com and lectures worldwide about the present crisis in our healthcare system and the affect it has on the doctor-patient relationship. This is Dr. Farrago's third book on direct primary care. *The Official Guide to Starting Your Own Direct Primary Care Practice* and *The Direct Primary Care Doctor's Daily Motivational Journal* are best sellers in this genre. He is a leading expert in direct primary care model and lectures medical students, residents and doctors on how to start their own DPC practice.

www.ingramcontent.com/pod-product-compliance
Lightning Source LLC
Chambersburg PA
CBHW030611270326
41927CB00007B/1126